Gut Ecology

Gut Ecology

Ailsa L Hart BMBCh MRCP
*Department of Gastroenterology, St Mark's Hospital,
London, UK*

Andrew J Stagg PhD
*Antigen Presentation Research Group, Faculty of
Medicine, Imperial College at Northwick Park
Hospital, London, UK*

Hans Graffner MD PhD
*Associate Professor and Medical Director,
Gastrointestinal Therapy Area, AstraZeneca
R & D Mölndal, Mölndal, Sweden*

Hans Glise MD PhD
*Associate Professor, Department of Surgery, Linköpings
University Hospital, and Head of Gastrointestinal
Therapy Area, AstraZeneca R & D Mölndal, Mölndal,
Sweden*

Per Falk MD PhD
*Associate Professor and Head of Molecular Biology,
AstraZeneca R & D Mölndal, Mölndal, Sweden*

Michael A Kamm MD FRACP FRCP
*Professor of Gastroenterology and Chairman of
Medicine, St Mark's Hospital, London, UK*

MARTIN DUNITZ

© 2002 Martin Dunitz Ltd, a member of the Taylor & Francis group

First published in the United Kingdom in 2002 by
Martin Dunitz Ltd
The Livery House
7–9 Pratt Street
London NW1 0AE
Tel: +44 (0)20 7482 2202
Fax: +44 (0)20 7267 0159
E-mail: info.dunitz@tandf.co.uk
Website: http://www.dunitz.co.uk

A CIP catalogue record for this book is available from the British Library

ISBN 1-84184-139-0

Distributed in the USA by Coventry University
Fulfilment Center
Taylor & Francis
7625 Empire Drive, Florence, KY 41042, USA
Toll Free Tel: +1 800 634 7064
E-mail: cserve@routledge_ny.com

Distributed in Canada by
Taylor & Francis
74 Rolark Drive
Scarborough, Ontario M1R 4G2, Canada
Toll Free Tel: +1 877 226 2237
E-mail: tal_fran@istar.ca

Distributed in the rest of the world by
ITPS Limited
Cheriton House, North Way
Andover, Hampshire SP10 5BE, UK
Tel: +44 (0)1264 332424
E-mail: reception@itps.co.uk

Front cover: Dr Kari Lounatmaa/Science Photo Library. **Phagocytosis** (coloured scanning electron micrograph of a polymorphonuclear leucocyte (orange) attacking *Bacillus cereus* bacteria (blue, rod-shaped)).

Printed and bound in Great Britain by The Cromwell Press, Trowbridge.

Contents

Contributors

S Peter Borriello
Director
Central Public Health Laboratory
61 Colindale Ave
London NW9 5HT, UK
Pborriello@PHLS.org.uk

Jonathan Braun
Professor and Chair
Department of Pathology and Laboratory
Medicine
UCLA School of Medicine CHS 13–222
Los Angeles, CA 90095–1732, USA
jbraun@mednet.ucla.edu

Massimo Campieri
Professor of Medicine &
Head of Inflammatory Bowel Disease Unit
Department of Internal Medicine and
Gastroenterology
Policlinico Sant'Orsola-Malpighi
Via Massarenti, 9
40138 Bologna, Italy
campieri@med.unibo.it

Kevin Collins
Associate Professor
Department of Microbiology & Medicine
University College
Cork, Ireland
microbiology@ucc.ie

Per Falk
Associate Professor &
Head of Molecular Biology
AstraZeneca R & D Mölndal
S-431 83 Mölndal, Sweden
per.falk@astrazeneca.com

Göte Forsberg
Departments of Clinical Sciences, Pediatrics,
and Clinical Microbiology, Immunology
Umeå University
S-901 85 Umeå, Sweden
gote.forsberg@pediatri.umu.se

Glenn R Gibson
Professor of Food Microbiology
Food Microbial Sciences Unit
Science and Technology Centre
University of Reading
Whiteknights
PO Box 226
Reading RG6 6AP, UK
g.r.gibson@reading.ac.uk

Paolo Gionchetti
IBD Unit
Department of Internal Medicine and
Gastroenterology
Policlinico Sant'Orsola-Malpighi
Via Massarenti 9
40138 Bologna, Italy
paolo@med.unibo.it

Hans Glise
Head of Gastrointestinal Therapy Area
AstraZeneca R & D Mölndal
S-431 83 Mölndal, Sweden
hans.glise@astrazeneca.com

Hans Graffner
Associate Professor and Medical Director
Gastroenterology Therapy Area
AstraZeneca R & D Mölndal
S-431 83 Mölndal, Sweden
hans.graffner@astrazeneca.com

Marie-Louise Hammarström
Department of Clinical Microbiology,
Immunology
Umeå University
S-901 85 Umeå, Sweden
marie-louise.hammarstrom@climi.umu.se

Sten Hammarström
Department of Clinical Microbiology,
Immunology
Umeå University
S-901 85 Umeå, Sweden
sten.hammarstrom@climi.umu.se

Ailsa L Hart
Department of Gastroenterology
St Mark's Hospital
Watford Road
Harrow HA1 3UJ, UK
ailsa.hart@btinternet.com

Olle Hernell
Professor of Paediatrics
Department of Clinical Sciences, Paediatrics
Umeå University
S-901 85 Umeå, Sweden
olle.hernell@pediatri.umu.se

Erika Isolauri
Professor of Paediatrics
Department of Paediatrics
University of Turku
20520 Turku, Finland
erika.isolauri@utu.fi

Anneli Ivarsson
Departments of Clinical Sciences, Pediatrics,
and Public Health and Clinical Medicine,
Epidemiology
Umeå University
S-901 85 Umeå, Sweden
anneli.ivarsson@epiph.umu.se

Martin F Kagnoff
Director Laboratory of Mucosal Immunology
University of California, San Diego
9500 Gilman Drive (MTF/412)
La Jolla, CA 92093–0623, USA
mkagnoff@ucsd.edu

Michael A Kamm
Professor of Gastroenterology and
Chairman of Medicine
St Mark's Hospital
Watford Road
Harrow HA1 3UJ, UK
kamm@ic.ac.uk

Alain Lamarre
Institute of Experimental Immunology
Universitätsspital
Schmelzbergstrasse 12
CH8091 Zürich, Switzerland
alamarre@pathol.unizh.ch

Thomas T MacDonald
Professor of Immunology
Director of the Division of Infection, Allergy,
Inflammation and Repair
Mailpoint 813
Level E, South Block
University of Southampton School of Medicine
Southampton SO16 6YD, UK
t.t.macdonald@soton.ac.uk

Andrew J Macpherson
Institute of Experimental Immunology
Universitätsspital
Schmelzbergstrasse 12
CH8091 Zürich, Switzerland
amacpher@pathol.unizh.ch

Tore Midtvedt
Laboratory of Medical Microbial Ecology
Karolinska Institute
Box 285
S-171 77 Stockholm, Sweden
Tore.Midtvedt@cmb.ki.se

Liam O'Mahony
Senior Research Scientist
National Food Biotechnology Centre
University College
Cork, Ireland
omahonyliam@yahoo.com

Giovanni Monteleone
Research Fellow
Division of Infection, Inflammation and Repair,
Mailpoint 813
Level E, South Block
University of Southampton School of Medicine
Southampton SO16 6YD, UK
g.monteleone@soton.ac.uk

Fernando Rizzello
IBD Unit
Department of Internal Medicine and
Gastroenterology
Policlinico Sant'Orsola-Malpighi
Via Massarenti, 9
40138 Bologna, Italy
fernandorizzello@hotmail.com

Seppo Salminen
Professor
Department of Biochemistry and Food
Chemistry
University of Turku
20014 Turku, Finland
sepsal@utu.fi

R Balfour Sartor
Professor of Medicine, Microbiology and
Immunology
Department of Medicine/Division of
Digestive Diseases
CB#7038 Room 032A Glaxo Building
Chapel Hill, NC 27599–7038, USA
rbs@med.unc.edu

Fergus Shanahan
Department of Medicine
University College
Cork, Ireland
f.shanahan@ucc.ie

Andrew J Stagg
Antigen Presentation Research Group
Imperial College School of Medicine
Northwick Park Institute of Medical Research
Watford Road
Harrow HA1 3UJ, UK
a.stagg@ic.ac.uk

Gerald W Tannock
Professor of Microbiology
Department of Microbiology
University of Otago
PO Box 56
700 Cumberland Street
Dunedin, New Zealand
gerald.tannock@stonebow.otago.ac.nz

Therese Uhr
Institute of Experimental Immunology
Universitätsspital
Schmelzbergstrasse 12
CH8091 Zürich, Switzerland
thuhr@pathol.unizh.ch

Preface

Lifelong cross-talk occurs between the host and the intestinal flora, and the outcome of this can determine whether health is maintained or disease intervenes. Our knowledge of the intestinal flora in health is limited. However, a combination of sophisticated molecular techniques, in conjunction with traditional microbiological methods, will pave the way for a greater understanding of this complex organ. This knowledge can then be used to explore disease prevention and treatment. An understanding of the bacteria-to-bacteria and bacteria-to-immune-cell interactions in the gastrointestinal tract will provide us with possible mechanisms of disease pathogenesis and potential ways of modulating the gastrointestinal microenvironment. In particular, under certain circumstances, the intestinal flora appears to have a role in driving inflammation. It remains to be seen which components of the flora are important in this process. Indeed, it may be that unique bacterial antigens are associated with disease in hosts with different genetic backgrounds.

Manipulating such a complex ecosystem is challenging. Therapeutic interventions are superimposed on a complex background with a high signal-to-noise ratio. Nonetheless, there is tantalising evidence from animal and human studies that such manipulation may be effective in treating disease. More evidence-based medicine is needed, but the proof of principle has led to a requirement to establish the mechanism of action, so that treatments can be targeted and other innovative approaches explored.

Ailsa L Hart
Andrew J Stagg
Hans Graffner
Hans Glise
Per Falk
Michael A Kamm

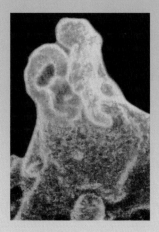

PART 1

The normal flora and techniques of identification

The normal flora of the gastrointestinal tract

S Peter Borriello

1

Introduction

There has been a re-emergence of interest in the interplay between the faecal microbiota, its associated metabolisms and its effect on gastrointestinal function. Much of the early interest was based on various hypotheses that linked gut bacterial metabolism of bile acids and ingested foodstuffs to the risk of developing colorectal and other cancers. Much of the current interest is fuelled by a re-emergence of recognition of the potential value of human and veterinary probiotics. An added stimulus in this area has been the relentless spread of antibiotic resistance.

A less widely known aspect of the interplay between gut bacteria and the host is the extent of involvement of commensal gastrointestinal bacteria in gut function, gut disease, and particularly disease of other organs. This should, however, be of little surprise when one considers that we each have about 10^{12} viable bacteria per gram of large bowel content, which is equivalent to more bacteria in our guts than there have ever been humans on the planet. To this quantitative complexity can be added a qualitative complexity of 400–500 different species. Consider the known metabolic capability of *Escherichia coli* alone: it is then immediately apparent that the metabolic capability of the gastrointestinal flora is immense, and surpasses that of the liver. In many respects, the gastrointestinal flora can be considered as a separate metabolic organ of the body. In fact, some of the less generally well-known aspects of this interplay between host and gastrointestinal flora relate to gut bacterial metabolites, for example, the production of volatile fatty acids that exacerbate acidaemias (such as methylmalonic acidaemia) and the associated role of antibiotics in patient management.[1] An area where there has been a resurgence of interest in the linkage between gut bacteria and cancer is the production of phyto-oestrogens from dietary precursors and their possible role in protection from, as opposed to induction of, hormone-dependent breast cancer.[2,3] The intriguing possibility of a role for such metabolites in infertility in humans remains unexplored. There is even evidence that gut bacteria can induce or repress liver cytochrome P450 owing to metabolism of dietary glucosinolates.[4]

There is a great deal of evidence that what is generally considered normal gut structure and function is, in fact, the end-point of a complex set of interactions between the host and microbes colonising the gut.[5] Such normal features include gastrointestinal motility, secretion and absorption, cell composition, mitotic activity, villous length, crypt depth, etc. More recently it has been shown that components of the gut microbiota can alter the colonic barrier function by modifying colonic wall permeability.[6] This interesting observation lends support to the hypothesis that increased intestinal permeability may be a key factor in the pathogenesis of idiopathic bowel disease, and that differences in the composition of the gut flora may contribute to this.

This chapter will concentrate on giving a broad description of the gastrointestinal flora at different sites, the main factors that control the flora at these sites, and some of the limitations on our ability to perform and/or interpret such studies.

Limitations to the study of the gastrointestinal flora

The microbial flora of the gastrointestinal tract forms an extremely complex ecosystem. There are at least 17 families of bacteria yielding at least 50 different genera. There are then countless species, subspecies and biotypes, with at least 400–500 different bacterial species thought to be present in the faecal flora of a single person.[7–9] This complexity imposes limitations on attempts to fully delineate the flora and changes in its composition. In order to interpret correctly the qualitative and quantitative data generated from studies on the flora of the gastrointestinal tract, it is important to be aware of the limitations imposed on such studies. The major problems are those of the complexity of the ecosystem and the inaccessibility of many parts of that ecosystem in a healthy subject. The difficulties that may influence the results fall into two major groups. First, sampling transport and storage, and, second cultivation, enumeration and identification.

Sampling, transport and storage

Obtaining specimens from any site other than the mouth and anus in healthy volunteers is difficult. However, even at these two sites there are issues to be considered. For example, analysis of porcine faecal material shows differences in the recoverable flora depending on from where in the stool specimen the sample is taken.[10] For parts of the gastrointestinal tract other than these sites, invasive techniques are employed (e.g. intubation), or collection of material at operation. This may lead to contamination of the specimen from other sites. In many cases the subject will have been anaesthetised and fasted, which both potentially have an effect on the flora. In particular, the reduction of peristalsis induced by anaesthetics will have an effect on the flora of the small bowel. Also, in many cases the subjects studied will have received antibiotics and/or a bowel washout.

The optimal collection vessel would be one in which an anaerobic atmosphere could be

maintained. In addition, the length of time the specimen remains in the collection vessel during transport will also influence the results. Further details of sampling and transport techniques are given in the review by Borriello *et al.*[11] If the specimen is not to be analysed immediately, then the length of time that it is stored prior to examination and the method of storage will also affect the recovery of bacteria. Even with a frequently used storage method[12] there are qualitative and quantitative changes in the flora, even after a relatively short storage time. If stored frozen, the rate of freezing and thawing of the specimen will also affect the bacteria present.[13]

Cultivation, enumeration and identification

A major problem in defining the flora of the gastrointestinal tract was the ability to cultivate the microorganisms present. This has been greatly overcome by the use of the polymerase chain reaction and direct sequence of 16S ribosomal DNA for molecular taxonomic studies of the flora.[14] However, such molecular approaches are not without limitations.[15] As the overwhelming majority of studies have used culture, and there is still merit in obtaining an isolate for further phenotypic, biochemical and genotypic analysis, it is worth considering some limitations of traditional culture. The most obvious is that the cultivation media used may not be able to support the growth of certain bacteria. So, although present and surviving transport and storage, they are not recovered. Others may grow slowly, and therefore the length of incubation, as well as the incubation conditions, are important variables. Few selective media are totally selective: some unwanted organisms may be isolated and some desired organisms will not be. For example, vancomycin, an antibiotic active against Gram-positive organisms, is frequently a component of selective media used for the isolation of bacteroides; however, some species of bacteroides are sensitive to this antibiotic.[16] Bacterial antagonism on culture media will also influence the recovery of bacteria.

Enumeration of bacteria may pose its own problems, a commonly overlooked one being the transfer of particulate material and associated bacteria through a dilution series. How the quantitative results are expressed also differs, e.g. triplicate or duplicate mean, or single analysis, or number per gram dry or wet weight of material. Also, the limit of detection is rarely stated and may vary from 10^2/g to 10^4/g between studies. 'Non-detected' therefore rarely means non-present, and should be interpreted differently between studies. This is more pronounced when studying biopsy material, where the amount of starting material can be very small and the limitation of detection in some studies as high as 10^6/g. Biopsy, or even operation, specimens for the study of mucosa-associated flora pose

problems of knowing how often to wash the material (and what wash fluid to use) to remove luminal flora 'contaminants' and not remove adherent mucosal flora.

Also, there is as yet no satisfactory way of expressing quantitative data for mucosa-adherent flora. To express it as per gram of tissue introduces variables of tissue thickness etc., but it is not yet possible to express accurately the number of bacteria per unit of surface area which would be much more meaningful. Another problem associated with enumeration is that of attempting to quantify individual species within a specimen. Even on selective media, less dominant species will be hidden within a confluent background of bacterial growth. On isolation media where discrete colonies are present, ideally every isolated colony present would have to be identified. This is rarely possible, and so, having isolated bacteria, three additional problems remain. What is a representative number of colonies to subculture for the purpose of identification? There is no good answer to this question other than 'as many as possible'. Once subcultured, viability must be retained, especially during storage if identification cannot be done immediately. The last problem is that of identification itself. This is now greatly facilitated by molecular taxonomic approaches. However, in the majority of the published literature, identification is based on familiarity and biochemical tests.

Microbial flora in different parts of the gastrointestinal tract

The composition of the flora within different parts of the gastrointestinal tract differs. In general (in health) from the stomach through to the colon there is a qualitative and quantitative increase in complexity. The exception to this is the oral flora, which is extremely complex.[17] A review of the flora at different sites and the key controlling mechanisms is to be found elsewhere.[18]

Stomach

In general it is considered that the healthy stomach is most often 'sterile' (i.e. fewer than 10^3 microorganisms/ml of content). Bacteria that are recovered tend to be Gram-positive. The most important factor controlling the flora within the stomach is acidity, with little evidence of a significant role for secretory immunoglobulin.[19] A more complex flora can be recovered following the ingestion of food and during conditions that result in a reduction of acidity,[20] for example achlorhydria due to hypogamma-globulinaemia.[19] The 'mucosal flora' of the stomach does not differ from that found in gastric juice,[19] with the possible exception of *Helicobacter pylori*.

Biliary tract

Aerobes are most frequently isolated from this site, but anaerobes can be isolated in up to 50% of culture-positive samples. The most frequently recovered anaerobes are *Clostridium perfringens* and *Bacteroides fragilis*.[21]

Proximal small bowel

The flora of the proximal small bowel (duodenum, jejunum and proximal ileum) is similar to that of the normal stomach, consisting predominantly of Gram-positive facultative bacteria, although enterobacteria and bacteroides can also be present. As in the stomach, the concentration of bacteria in the jejunum can increase soon after a meal,[20] and generally in the small bowel in subjects with hypochlorhydria.[20,22] The key factor controlling the flora in the small bowel is peristalsis, and factors that compromise this can lead to small bowel overgrowth. Duodenal juice has antibacterial activity,[23] but its significance is still to be determined. The role of natural antibodies in controlling the flora at this site is also uncertain, with little evidence of small bowel overgrowth in immunodeficient patients, or of significant differences compared with control subjects.[24] There has been little published work on the nature of the mucosal flora in the proximal small bowel, and what has been done has shown it to be essentially the same as the luminal flora.[25]

Distal small bowel

In both the distal and terminal ileum the complexity of the flora starts to approach that of the large bowel, with a marked shift towards Gram-negative bacteria and anaerobes compared to the proximal small bowel. As in the proximal small bowel, immunodeficiency appears to have little effect on the composition of the flora.[24]

Large bowel

The large bowel is the most heavily colonised part of the gastrointestinal tract. Most work on the bacterial flora has concentrated on the analysis of faecal specimens, with much less information being available on the flora of the caecum and appendix, or that associated with the mucosa. In general, it would appear that the flora of the large intestine is qualitatively similar to that of faeces.[8,26,27] In animal studies the caecal and faecal flora has been shown to be the same for the rat and mouse, but for the rabbit and guinea pig a number of differences are evident.[28] It would appear that the flora of the appendix may be different from that of other areas of the colon.[29] However, these possible differences must be treated with caution, as the results were derived from material from patients at operation and may not reflect the flora in health. A number of factors have been proposed as being involved in the control of the microbial flora of the

large bowel. Of these, microbial interference, both cooperative and antagonistic, plays a major role. This is probably best exemplified by the exertion of colonisation resistance to implantation by 'foreign' commensals or pathogens, e.g. *Clostridum difficile*.[30] The role of the other factors proposed as being involved in the control of the large bowel flora is much more difficult to determine. This is predominantly because attempts to monitor the effects of different factors have depended on microbial analysis of the faecal flora, which does not necessarily reflect changes occurring elsewhere in the large bowel. Of these factors, diet has probably received the most attention. The reasons for this are twofold. First, it is the factor that is most easily manipulated, and second, there is a great deal of interest in the possible interrelationships between diet, gastrointestinal flora and disease, especially large bowel cancer. In general it has been difficult to show significant changes in the faecal flora after feeding volunteers different diets. However, some changes have been noted. Overall, a high-carbohydrate diet is associated with an increase in bifidobacteria, a high-fat diet with an increase in bacteroides, and an elemental diet with a decrease in enterococci and lactobacilli. Greater changes in response to diet are detected when measuring changes in the metabolic capability of the flora. For example, an elemental diet in humans leads to decreases in the metabolism of cholesterol and bile acid and the production of phenols. A high-beef diet in rats leads to increases in β-glucuronidase, nitroreductase and azoreductase, and a decrease in β-glucosidase activity.

Although bacteria can cause diarrhoea, it is also true that diarrhoea-related changes in the gut environment affect the gut flora. For example, there is a 10^5-fold reduction in bacteroides in the faeces of patients with cholera.[31] Induction of diarrhoea by a peroral saline perfusion of the terminal ileum resulted in an increase in faecal coliforms[32] whereas the use of lactulose[33] or cascara and milk of magnesia[34] resulted in an overall decrease in coliforms and enterococci.

As expected there is much less published work on the mucosal flora of the large bowel than on the faecal flora. In general, the evidence is that, qualitatively, the mucosal flora differs little from luminal flora, but the ratio and total numbers of different genera differ. For example, anaerobes appear to be less dominant at mucosal surfaces, with ratios of total anaerobes to aerobes ranging from 1:1 to 10^4:1, but generally close to 2:1.[35–37] Very few studies report on differences in the mucosal flora at different large bowel sites within the same patient, and some report little overall detected difference, e.g. for *Escherichia coli*[38] while some report observations on differences for specific species, e.g. lactobacilli, megasphaera, acidaminococci and veillonella,[39] staphylococci[37] and clostridia.[18]

Work on following the development of the gastrointestinal flora in humans has been restricted to analysis of the faecal flora. In the 1970s there was much interest in monitoring the development of the faecal flora during the first few weeks of life, and in particular the effect on the faecal flora of feeding breast milk or infant formula. This was one situation where diet had a major measurable effect, such as lower concentrations of bifidobacteria and higher concentrations of *Escherichia coli* and putrefactive clostridia in the faeces of formula milk-fed infants, and the converse in breast milk-fed infants.[40] As the composition of formula feed has changed (e.g. lower buffering capacity) the differences in faecal flora readily apparent in the past have become less evident.

Succession, in broad terms, is that facultatives colonise first and probably create conditions that are favourable for the establishment of anaerobes, owing to reduction of the redox potential. The first anaerobes to colonise are clostridia (e.g. *C. perfringens* and *C. tertium*), and these are also the first anaerobes to be detected (not to be confused with colonisation), which probably reflects spores passing through the gut. Bifidobacteria are also early anaerobe colonisers. The flora becomes immensely more complex at weaning, and starts to exhibit colonisation resistance at this stage.[41]

What is normal?

Most gut flora studies are undertaken on western subjects. Further, gut material other than faeces is rarely analysed in healthy individuals, such materials consisting of resected tissue distant from a tumour at operation, or an extra biopsy, or gastric and other juices sampled during examination of the patient. Most such analyses are therefore conducted on material from subjects with known or presumed underlying conditions, who may be on medication, or who received anaesthetics or pre- or perioperative antibiotics. Even those studies undertaken on sudden-death victims, such as road traffic casualties, suffer from not considering the medical history of the subject (they may have been taking antibiotics for a respiratory tract infection) and our ignorance of changes in the flora that may occur *post mortem*.

Two examples highlight the problem of making generalisations based on results from western subjects. First, although gastric anacidity is rare in young people in Northern Europe and North America, it is not uncommon in other parts of the world, e.g. South America.[42] It may be possible that gastric colonisation is a more common state of affairs when viewed on a worldwide basis. Second, a more profuse proximal small bowel flora is found in India,[43,44] consisting predominantly of Gram-positive aerobic and anaerobic cocci.

Conclusions

The microbial ecology of the gut is still very poorly understood, in terms of both composition and function, and factors that may alter the flora. Much of what has been published over the last 40 years must be interpreted with caution. There is little doubt that the increasing activity in this field of interest and the concomitant application of increasingly sophisticated science, will offer a better understanding of what is normal and what is abnormal. It will indicate possible beneficial interventions, as well as provide new insights into the complex interplay between the host and its microbiota.

References

1. Bain MD, Jones M, Borriello SP, *et al.* Contribution of gut bacterial metabolism to human metabolic disease. *Lancet* 1988; 1: 1078–1079.

2. Setchell KDR, Borriello SP, Hulme P, *et al.* Non-steroidal oestrogens of dietary origin: Possible roles in hormone dependent disease. *Am J Clin Nutr* 1984; 40:569–578.

3. Ingram D, Sanders K, Kolybaba M, Lopez D. Case-control study of phyto-oestrogens and breast cancer. *Lancet* 1997; 350:990–994.

4. Nugon-Baudon L, Robot S, Flinois JP, *et al.* Effects of the bacterial status of rats on the changes in some liver cytochrome P450 (EC 1.14.14.1) apoproptein consequent to a glucosinolate-rich diet. *Br J Nutr* 1998; 80:231–234.

5. Borriello SP, Bacteria and gastrointestinal secretion and motility. *Scand J Gastroenterol* 1984; 19(Suppl 93):115–121.

6. Garcia-Lafuent A, Antolin M, Guarner F, *et al.* Modulations of colonic barrier function by

the composition of the commensal flora in the rat. *Gut* 2001; 48:503–507.

7. Moore WEC, Holdeman LV. Human fecal flora: the normal flora of 20 Japanese-Hawaiians. *Appl Microbiol* 1974; 27: 961–979.

8. Moore WEC, Holdeman LV. Discussion of current bacteriological investigations of the relationships between intestinal flora, diet and colon cancer, *Cancer Res* 1975; 35:3418–3420.

9. Moore WEC, Holdeman LV. Some newer concepts of the human intestinal flora. *Am J Med Technol* 1975; 41:427–430.

10. Rall GD, Wood AJ, Wescott RB, Dommert AR. Distribution of bacteria in feces of swine. *Appl Microbiol* 1970; 20:789–792.

11. Borriello SP, Hudson M, Hill M. Investigation of the gastrointestinal bacteria flora. In: Russell RI, ed. *Clinics in Gastroenterology*, Vol. 7. Philadelphia: WB Saunders, 1978; 329–349.

12. Crowther JS. Transport and storage of faeces for bacteriological examination. *J App Bacteriol* 1971; 34:477–483.

13. Calcott PH, Lee SK, MacLeod RA. The effect of cooling and warming rates on the survival of a variety of bacteria. *Can J Microbiol* 1976; 22:106–109.

14. Wilson KH, Blitchington RB. Human colonic biota studied by ribosomal DNA sequence analysis. *Appl Environ Microbiol* 1996; 62: 2273–2278.

15. O'Sullivan DJ Methods for analysis of the intestinal microflora. In: Tannock GW, ed. *Probiotics: a critical review*. Dunedin: Horizon Scientific Press, 1999; 23–44.

16. van Winkelhoff AJ, De Graff J. Vancomycin as a selective agent for isolation of Bacteroides species. *J Clin Microbiol* 1983; 18:1282–1284.

17. Marsh P. The normal oral flora. In: March P, *Oral Microbiology*. Aspects of Microbiology Series. Surrey: Nelson, 1980; 11–24.

18. Borriello SP. Microbial flora of the gastrointestinal tract. In: Hill MJ, ed. *Microbial Metabolisms in the Digestive Tract*. Florida: CRC Press Inc, 1986; 1–19.

19. Dolby JM, Webster ADG, Borriello SP, *et al.* Bacterial colonization and nitrite concentration in the achlorhydric stomachs of patients with primary hypogammaglobulinaemia or classical pernicious anaemia. *Scand J Gastroenterol* 1984; 19:105–110.

20. Drasar BS, Shiner M, McLeod GM. Studies on the intestinal flora. 1. The bacterial flora of the gastrointestinal tract in healthy and achlorhydric persons. *Gastroenterology* 1969; 56:71–79.

21. Sakaguchi Y, Murata K, Kimura M. *Clostridium perfringens* and other anaerobes isolated from bile. *J Clin Pathol* 1983; 36: 345–349.

22. Drasar BS, Shiner M. Studies on the intestinal flora. II. Bacterial flora of the small intestine in patients with gastrointestinal disorders. *Gut* 1969; 10:812–819.

23. Umenai T, Sasaki T, Konno T. Antibacterial activity detected in duodenal juice. *Tohoku J Exp Med* 1977; 122:299–300.

24. Brown WR, Savage DC, Dubois RS, *et al.* Intestinal microflora of immunoglobulin-deficient and normal human subjects. *Gastroenterology* 1972; 62:1143–1152.

25. Plaut AG, Gorbach SL, Nahas L, *et al.* Studies of intestinal microflora. III. The microbial flora of human small intestinal mucosa and fluids. *Gastroenterology* 1967; 53: 868–873.

26. Moore WEC, Cato EP, Holdeman LV.

Anaerobic bacteria of the gastrointestinal flora and their occurrence in clinical infections. *J Infect Dis* 1969; 119:641–649.

27. Gorbach SL, Plaut AG, Nahas L, *et al.* Studies of intestinal microflora. II. Micro-organisms of the small intestine and their relations to oral and fecal flora. *Gastroenterology* 1967; 53: 856–867.

28. Hawksworth GM, Drasar BS, Hill MJ. Intestinal bacteria and the hydrolysis of glycosidic bonds. *J Med Microbiol* 1971; 4:451–459.

29. Seeliger H, Werner H. Recherches qualitatives et quantitatives sur la flore intestinale de l'homme. *Ann Inst Pasteur* 1963; 105:911–936.

30. Borriello SP, Barclay FE. Anaerobes in intestinal homeostasis. In: Duerden BI, Drasar BS, eds. *Anaerobes in Human Disease.* London: Edward Arnold, 1990; 343–350.

31. Gorbach SL, Banwell JG, Jacobs B, *et al.* Intestinal microflora in Asiatic cholera. I. 'Rice-water' stool. *J Infect Dis* 1970; 121: 33–37.

32. Gorbach SL, Nahas L, Plant AG, *et al.* Studies of intestinal microflora. V. Fecal microbial ecology in ulcerative colitis and regional enteritis: relationship to severity of disease and chemotherapy. *Gastroenterology* 1968; 54: 575–587.

33. Haenel HW, Fedheim W, Muller-Beuthow W, Rutloff H. Versuche zur unstimmung der faecalen flora des gesunden erwachsenen. *Zbl Bakt* 1958; 188:70–80.

34. Levison ME, Kaye D. Fecal flora in man: effect of cathartic. *J Infect Dis* 1969; 119: 591–596.

35. Croucher SC, Houston AP, Bayliss CE, Turner RJ. Bacterial populations associated with different regions of the human colon wall. *Appl Environ Microbiol* 1983; 45: 1025–1033.

36. Peach S, Lock MR, Katz D, *et al.* Mucosal-associated bacterial flora of the intestine in patients with Crohn's disease and in a control group. *Gut* 1978; 19:1034–1042.

37. Nelson DP, Mata LJ. Bacterial flora associated with the human gastrointestinal mucosa. *Gastroenterology* 1970; 58:56–61.

38. Hartley CL, Neumann CS, Richmond MH. Adhesion of commensal bacteria to the large intestine wall in humans. *Infect Immun* 1979; 23:128–132.

39. Edmiston CE Jr, Avant GR, Wilson FA. Anaerobic bacterial populations on normal and diseased human biopsy tissue. *Appl Environ Microbiol* 1982; 43:1173–1181.

40. Borriello SP, Stephens S. The development of the infant gut flora and the medical microbiology of infant botulism and necrotizing enterocolitis. In: Goodwin, CS ed. *Microbes and Infections of the Gut.* London: Blackwell Scientific, 1984; 1–26.

41. Borriello SP, Barclay FE. An *in vitro* model of colonisation resistance to *Clostridium difficile* infection. *J Med Microbiol* 1986; 21:299–309.

42. Correa P, Coello C, Duque E. Carcinoma and intestinal metaplasia of the stomach in Colombian migrants. *J Natl Cancer Inst* 1970; 44:297–306.

43. Bhat P, Shantakumari S, Rajan D, *et al.* Bacterial flora of the gastrointestinal tract in Southern Indian control subjects and patients with tropical sprue. *Gastroenterology* 1972; 62:11–21.

44. Bhat P, Albert MJ, Rajan D, *et al.* Bacterial flora of the jejunum: a comparison of luminal aspirate and mucosal biopsy. *J Med Microbiol* 1980; 13:247–256.

The gut microflora: traditional and molecular identification techniques

Gerald W Tannock

2

Culture and phenotype: tradition

Much of our knowledge of the composition of the gut
microflora in humans is derived from bacteriological studies
that used the traditional techniques of culture, microscopy
and the determination of the fermentative and other
biochemical capabilities of bacterial isolates. This work, still
important in studies of the microflora, requires the use of
apparatus such as anaerobic glove boxes, or test tubes flushed
with an oxygen-free gas, to provide a suitably reduced
environment that will enable extremely oxygen-sensitive
bacteria to be cultivated. The numerically predominant
members of the microflora are obligate anaerobic bacteria,
and perhaps hundreds of species may be capable of inhabiting
the human intestinal tract. The logistics associated with the
isolation and identification of obligate anaerobic bacteria are
thus formidable. In the end, one must also admit that the
success of phenotypic identification methods often relies on
the experience of the laboratory worker and a dose of
intuition. This is because there is considerable intraspecies
variation with regard to biochemical properties. In addition,
phenotypic characteristics are readily influenced by the

culture conditions under which the bacteria are maintained and tested. Nevertheless, a vote of gratitude is due to the pioneers of anaerobic bacteriology (Veillon, Prevot, Hungate, Holdeman and Moore, Sutter and Finegold and their respective colleagues) who developed relatively rational and effective identification systems for obligate anaerobic gut bacteria.[1-6]

Culture and genotype: phylogeny

Carl Woese[7] revealed that small ribosomal subunit RNA (16S rRNA in the case of bacteria) contained regions of nucleotide base sequence that were highly conserved, and that these were interspersed with hypervariable regions (V regions). These hypervariable regions contained the signatures of phylogenetic groups and even species. Members of the gut microflora can be accurately identified by extraction of DNA from a pure culture of a bacterial isolate, polymerase chain reaction (PCR) amplification of the 16S rRNA gene using universal primers that target conserved sequences, and determination of its nucleotide base sequence. For utmost accuracy, the whole gene (about 1500 bp) should be sequenced, but a sequence of 500 bp will provide useful information. The sequence can be compared with those available in gene databanks in order to determine the closest match, and

hence an identification of the bacterial isolate. There are currently about 16,000 16S rRNA gene sequences stored by the ribosomal database project II, for example, although not all are of complete genes. Doubtless there are intestinal species that are still not represented in gene databanks. 16S rRNA gene sequences can be used to construct phylogenetic trees of the members of the intestinal microflora. This contributes greatly to bacterial taxonomy. Molecular taxonomy provides a concrete basis for the identification of bacterial species. A sequence of As, Ts, Gs and Cs is tangible and not influenced by the cultivation conditions to which the bacteria have been subjected. The pioneers in the identification of human intestinal bacteria by 16S rRNA gene sequencing must surely be Wilson and Blitchington.[8]

Culture and genotype: denaturing gradient gel electrophoresis

For the microbiologist faced with identifying hundreds of bacterial isolates, PCR amplification and whole gene sequencing may not be regarded as essential. Indeed, some microbial ecologists may view modern studies of the faecal microflora as 'death by phylogeny'. PCR amplification of short sequences of 16S rDNA that are hypervariable can provide a rapid identification method when coupled with denaturing gradient gel electrophoresis (DGGE). In PCR/DGGE, fragments of the 16S rRNA gene (no more than 400 bp in length) are amplified by PCR. One of the primers has a GC-rich 5' end (GC clamp) to prevent complete denaturation of the DNA fragments. The double-stranded 16S fragments migrate through a polyacrylamide gel containing a gradient of urea and formamide until they are partially denatured by the chemical conditions. The fragments do not denature completely because of the GC clamp, and migration is radically slowed when partial denaturation occurs. Because of the variation in the 16S sequences of different bacterial species, chemical stability is also different; therefore, different 16S 'species' can be differentiated by this electrophoretic method.[9] The V2–V3 region of the 16S rRNA gene, for example, can be amplified from pure cultures of *Lactobacillus* isolates. The PCR amplicons, when examined by DGGE, allow the identification of many *Lactobacillus* species because their V2–V3 sequences have characteristic migration properties in the electrophoretic gel. This means that an identification ladder can be prepared from type cultures in order to identify isolates of intestinal lactobacilli.[10] This approach has also been found to be appropriate for the identification of *Bacteroides* and *Bifidobacterium* species (Munro and Tannock, unpublished) and is doubtless applicable to many other bacterial genera.

Culture and genotype: species-specific PCR primers

Hypervariable regions of the 16S rRNA gene also provide targets for the derivation of genus- and species-specific PCR primers. Numerous examples already exist in the scientific literature, but those useful in the identification of bifidobacteria can be cited here. Matsuki and Tanaka[11] have reported PCR primer sets that will differentiate between nine bifidobacterial species (*B. catenulatum* and *B. pseudocatenulatum* cannot be differentiated from each other). This is an outstanding accomplishment, considering the high degree of similarity in 16S rRNA gene sequences of the members of this genus.[12] Targets for species-specific primers may be found elsewhere on the bacterial chromosome. PCR primers that anneal to conserved sequences in the 16S and 23S rRNA genes of lactobacilli, for example, allowed the amplification of DNA between these two genes (intergenic spacer region).[13] A high degree of hypervariability of the spacer region was observed, and this permitted the derivation of primers that target these sequences and differentiate between *Lactobacillus* species. Eight primer sets that target the intergenic spacer region sequence for the identification of *Lactobacillus* species are currently available.[10] The use of primer sets to identify bacterial species is logistically demanding and expensive. For example, consider the requirements to test each bifidobacterial isolate in nine separate PCR reactions to achieve identification. Probably the best use of species-specific primers is in the confirmation of the results obtained by identification methods such as PCR/DGGE, and in the direct detection of species, without culture, in faecal or intestinal samples.

Culture and genotype: genetic fingerprinting

The identification techniques described thus far are aimed at the identification of bacterial species. The latter, however, can be further divided into strains using molecular typing methods. These typing methods are generally based on restriction fragment length polymorphisms of bacterial DNA. Restriction endonuclease digests of DNA extracted from pure bacterial cultures are analysed by agarose gel electrophoresis. The resulting patterns of DNA fragments are characteristic of each strain. Ribotyping and pulsed-field gel electrophoresis (PFGE) of DNA digests are examples of methods that have been used to differentiate between strains of intestinal bacteria.[14,15] Such methodologies are extremely useful in tracking the fate of specific bacterial strains in the intestinal ecosystem, just as they are in studying the epidemiology of bacterial pathogens. An important observation resulting from the use of molecular typing concerns *Lactobacillus*–host

relationships. Genetic fingerprinting of bacterial isolates was used to analyse the composition of the *Lactobacillus* populations present in the faeces of humans during a study aimed at measuring the impact of probiotic consumption on the composition of the faecal microflora. The composition of the faecal microflora of 10 healthy subjects was monitored before (control period of 6 months), during (test period of 6 months) and after (post-test period of 3 months) the administration of a milk product containing *Lactobacillus rhamnosus* DR20 (daily dose of 1.6×10^9 lactobacilli). The composition of the *Lactobacillus* population of each subject was analysed by PFGE of bacterial DNA digests in order to differentiate between DR20 and other strains present in the samples. Consumption of the probiotic altered the composition of the *Lactobacillus* populations of the subjects, but to varying degrees. The presence of DR20 among the numerically predominant strains was related to the presence or absence of a stable autochthonous population of lactobacilli during the control period. The probiotic strain did not predominate in samples collected from subjects with *Lactobacillus* populations of stable composition. The presence of lactobacilli capable of persisting long term (autochthonous strains) in the faeces of a subject appeared to preclude the establishment of DR20 (allochthonous) as the numerically dominant strain.[16]

No culture: just genotype

The culture of bacteria is a prerequisite to the foregoing identification methods. About 60% of the intestinal microflora is, however, non-cultivable even when excellent anaerobic culture methods are employed. This means that many of the intestinal inhabitants have never been studied in the laboratory. Methods based on bacterial nucleic acids overcome this problem because cultivation of the bacteria is not necessary. As shown by the pioneering work of Zoetendal, Akkermans and De Vos,[17] bacterial DNA can be extracted directly from intestinal or faecal samples. Hypervariable 16S rDNA sequences can be amplified using universal PCR primers. The mixture of hypervariable DNA fragments can be separated by DGGE, and a profile of 90–99% of the bacterial community is generated. Individual fragments of DNA can be cut from DGGE gels, further amplified and cloned, and then sequenced. The sequence can be compared with those in gene databanks in order to identify the bacterium from which the 16S sequence originated. Depending on the length of the sequence, at least the bacterial phylogenetic group can be identified. In a further development of this methodology, PCR primers specific for bacterial groups can be derived. These primers generate a DGGE profile of the species comprising a specific bacterial group within the bacterial community.[18]

In a period of about 30 years, the identification of intestinal bacteria has developed from 'culture and phenotype' to 'no culture, just genotype'. For those who regret the passing of almost total reliance on bacteriological culture for analysis of the gut microflora, and the feel of agar beneath their fingernails, future research will probably still require the cultivation and identification of at least some members of the bacterial community. In order to understand the pathogenesis of inflammatory conditions of the bowel, for example, fulfilment of Koch's postulates (perhaps in modified form) will doubtless be necessary with regard to particular groups within the gut microflora. This work will require the cultivation and identification of specific bacteria in order to derive the defined experimental animal systems that are required for this work.

References

1. Finegold SM, Attebery HR, Sutter VL. Effect of diet on human fecal flora: comparison of Japanese and American diets. *Am J Clin Nutr* 1974; 27:1456–1469.

2. Finegold SM, Sutter VL. Fecal flora in different populations, with special reference to diet. *Am J Clin Nutr* 1978; 31:S116–S122.

3. Holdeman LV, Moore WEC. *Anaerobe Laboratory Manual* 2nd edn. Blacksburg: VPI Anaerobe Laboratory, 1973.

4. Moore WE, Cato EP, Holdeman LV. Some current concepts in intestinal bacteriology. *Am J Clin Nutr* 1978; 31:S33–42.

5. Moore WE, Holdeman LV. Special problems associated with the isolation and identification of intestinal bacteria in fecal flora studies. *Am J Clin Nutr* 1974; 27:1450–1455.

6. Summanen P, Baron EJ, Citron DM, *et al. Wadsworth Anaerobic Bacteriology Manual* 5th edn. Belmont: Star Publishing Company, 1993.

7. Woese CR. Bacterial evolution. *Microbiol Rev* 1987; 51:221–271.

8. Wilson KH, Blitchington RB. Human colonic biota studied by ribosomal DNA sequence analysis. *Appl Environ Microbiol* 1996; 62: 2273–2278.

9. Muyzer G, Smalla K. Application of denaturing gradient gel electrophoresis (DGGE) and temperature gradient gel electrophoresis (TGGE) in microbial ecology. *Antonie Van Leeuwenhoek* 1998; 73:127–141.

10. Walter J, Tannock GW, Tilsala-Timisjarvi A, *et al.* Detection and identification of gastrointestinal *Lactobacillus* species by using denaturing gradient gel electrophoresis and species-specific PCR primers. *Appl Environ Microbiol* 2000; 66:297–303.

11. Matsuki T, Watanabe K, Tanaka R, *et al.* Distribution of bifidobacterial species in human intestinal microflora examined with 16S rRNA-gene-targeted species-specific primers. *Appl Environ Microbiol* 1999; 65: 4506–4512.

12. Leblond-Bourget N, Philippe H, Mangin I, Decaris B. 16S rRNA and 16S to 23S internal transcribed spacer sequence analyses reveal inter- and intraspecific *Bifidobacterium* phylogeny. *Int J Syst Bacteriol* 1996; 46: 102–111.

13. Tannock GW, Tilsala-Timisjarvi A, Rodtong S, *et al.* Identification of *Lactobacillus* isolates from the gastrointestinal tract, silage, and yoghurt by 16S-23S rRNA gene intergenic spacer region sequence comparisons. *Appl Environ Microbiol* 1999; 65:4264–4267.

14. Kimura K, McCartney AL, McConnell MA, Tannock GW. Analysis of fecal populations of bifidobacteria and lactobacilli and investigation of the immunological responses of their human hosts to the predominant strains. *Appl Environ Microbiol* 1997; 63: 3394–3398.

15. McCartney AL, Wenzhi W, Tannock GW. Molecular analysis of the composition of the bifidobacterial and lactobacillus microflora of humans. *Appl Environ Microbiol* 1996; 62: 4608–4613.

16. Tannock GW, Munro K, Harmsen HJM, *et al.* Analysis of the fecal microflora of human subjects consuming a probiotic containing *Lactobacillus rhamnosus* DR20. *Appl Environ Microbiol* 2000; 66:2578–2588.

17. Zoetendal EG, Akkermans AD, De Vos WM. Temperature gradient gel electrophoresis analysis of 16S rRNA from human fecal samples reveals stable and host-specific communities of active bacteria. *Appl Environ Microbiol* 1998; 64:3854–3859.

18. Satokari RM, Vaughan EE, Akkermans ADL, *et al.* Bifidobacterial diversity in human feces detected by genus-specific PCR and denaturing gradient gel electrophoresis. *Appl Environ Microbiol* 2001; 67:504–513.

The gut microflora: functional identification techniques

Jonathan Braun and Bo Wei

3

Introduction

Normal mucosal homeostasis is the interdependent relationship of epithelium, luminal microorganisms and the regional immune system.[1,2] The mammalian immune system has an exceptional capacity for specific antigen recognition and immunologic memory to microbial antigens, and for powerful amplification of effector mechanisms against such antigenic targets.[3] These properties obviously require special adaptation to preserve the mucosal–microbial interrelationship essential for normal intestinal function.

It is widely understood that inflammatory bowel disease (IBD) involves a chronic disturbance in this homeostasis. In recent years, there has been a particular effort to understand this homeostatic disturbance in the context of immunologic activation and tissue damage.[4,5] In particular, this effort has been informed by the emerging understanding of *Helicobacter pylori* pathogenesis in peptic ulcer disease. From this, we have learned that the manifestation of clinical disease reflects the interplay of commensal bacterial and host traits. Together, these affect levels of colonization and the nature and intensity of inflammation and tissue damage.[6,7] Intestinal microorganisms are diverse, and the majority are difficult or impossible to culture. Thus, it is a major challenge to identify those with pertinent traits eliciting such responses in susceptible hosts.

This challenge requires screening and isolation strategies that center on the *functional* properties of a candidate microbial population. Three major approaches have emerged, each facilitated by recombinant and genomic experimental strategies (Table 3.1).

High-throughput phylogenetic identification

The intestinal microbiota comprises a highly complex population and has classically been characterized by demanding and fastidious microbiologic culture strategies.[8] However, such procedures are unsuitable for high-throughput analysis in experimental and population studies, and perhaps 40% of the microbial residents are non-culturable. This situation has been resolved to a significant extent by the introduction of 16S rDNA polymorphism analysis.[9,10] In particular, the conceptual and technologic innovations of Tannock and colleagues[11] have permitted the application of this strategy to quantitative and high-throughput analysis (see Chapter 2 in this volume).

We anticipate two technologies that may further advance phylogenetic analysis. First, high-density DNA microarrays may offer an appealing alternative platform for PCR/DGGE analysis of 16S rDNA

Table 3.1
Functional identification of gut microbiota

Strategy	Analyte	Technology
High-throughput phylogenetics	16S rDNA	DNAChip Real-time PCR (Taqman)
Expression cloning	Antibody targets Enzymes	Bacterial expression cloning
Subtractive cloning	Genes of distinctive abundance, localization	Genomic representational difference analysis (RDA) cDNA suppression subtractive hybridization (SSH) Differential display hybridization (DDH)

phylogenetics. The advantage is the simplicity of wet analysis using, in principle, a single 16S rDNA PCR product to probe a DNA chip with hundreds of species-specific oligonucleotides. The two challenges to overcome are validated single specificity and reproducibility; and the small dynamic range of DNA chips (~ 2 logs), which may impair the assessment of minor components of the bacterial population. However, it is also conceivable that new targets besides 16S rDNA may emerge for phylogenetic or functional definition of bacterial populations. Such targets would be most easily introduced in this format.

Secondly, real-time PCR (RT-PCR) permits remarkably quantitative assessment of mRNA levels with a very large dynamic substrate range (4–5 logs).[12] When coupled with semi-automated microtiter plate format, this converts RT-PCR to a true high-throughput quantitative assay system. Like DNA microarray, this technology is very flexible for target analysis.

Expression cloning

Functional definition of bacterial populations has primarily involved immunochemical strategies. Disordered mucosal environments are associated with antibody responses to local immunogenic microbial species cells.[13] These antibodies can be useful reagents to identify microorganisms participating in the

disordered environment. The analytic use of conventional serum antibodies can be hampered by the complexity of serum antibody specificities, the low titer of such antibodies, and the heterogeneity of different donors. This problem is largely overcome by the production of monoclonal antibodies. Initially, hybridomas offered the sole strategy for monoclonal antibody creation, but more recently, phage display technology has offered a second option. In this method, immunoglobulin genes from populations of antigen-reactive B cells are molecularly cloned, and expressed in large recombinant libraries using a phage vector. Such vectors are constructed such that a Fab or Fv antibody binding site is expressed as a surface protein on the phage particle. In this fashion, such libraries create phage populations directly selectable for a binding specificity. In addition, bacterial expression systems provide rapid, large-scale antibody production. Together, these features permit efficient isolation and production of representative marker antibodies for analytic and preparative applications.[14–17]

With such reagents, the second half of the task emerges: the isolation and identification of microbial antigens. Typically, this has depended on microbiologic culture of candidate bacterial populations, and filter-based probing for immunoreactive proteins (such as colony lifts and Western analysis). An example of this approach was our isolation (by phage display) of an IBD-associated marker antibody, and its use in the identification of immunoreactive colonic bacteria species. Through a process of microbiologic cloning, protein microsequencing, and molecular cloning, the resulting proteins were identified and subsequently immunologically associated with Crohn's disease (CD).[18–20]

An important limitation of immunochemical strategies in microbial discovery is that organisms are often uncommon, fastidious or unculturable. However, recent advances in recombinant expression cloning raise the possibility of a much more flexible and potentially powerful approach to bacterial population analysis. In particular, PCR-based exon trapping offers a simple method for the production of highly diverse expression cloning of bacterial populations. When coupled with protein microarrays, such libraries may permit high-throughput identification and isolation of microbial antigen with immunochemical reagents. Moreover, this technology also permits the search for proteins with other functionally important characteristics, such as enzymatic or receptor/ligand activity.[21,22]

Third, subtractive cloning, notably representational difference analysis, can identify unique sequences reflecting microorganisms distinguished by distinctive abundance or localization. Coupled with accumulating microbial genome databases, such sequences can point to candidate microorganisms for isolation and functional assessment. Subtractive cloning is exemplified by the isolation of a novel bacterial gene, PFTR (formerly, I2), in CD lesion mucosa versus adjacent uninvolved mucosa. This sequence represented a novel tetR family bacterial transcription factor which, through genomic homolog evaluation, was found to originate from *Pseudomonas fluorescens*. Quantitative PCR established that the PFTR(I2) sequence reflects an apparent commensal colonization of the ileum, but a pathologic colonization of the colon in CD. Antibody levels to this protein are disease associated; in the mouse, PFTR protein by several lines of evidence is a T-cell superantigen, and elicits a strong IFNγ response in colitis-susceptible mouse strains. These findings indicate that PFTR and *Ps. fluorescens*, identified by a subtractive cloning strategy, are likely to illuminate microbial pathogenesis in CD.[15,23–26]

These approaches and examples demonstrate the wave of high-throughput genomic and expression methods for microbial characterization. They also reflect new challenges for hypothesis formation and biologic validation.

References

1. Zinkernagel RM, Bachmann MF, Kundig TM, *et al.* On immunological memory. *Annu Rev Immunol* 1996; 14:333–367.

2. Wren BW. Microbial genome analysis: insights into virulence, host adaption, and evolution. *Nature Genet* 2000; 1:30–39.

3. Hoffmann JAF, Kafatos C, Janeway CA, Ezekowitz RAB. Phylogenetic perspectives in innate immunity. *Science* 1999; 284: 1313–1318.

4. Martin HM, Rhodes JM. Bacteria and inflammatory bowel disease. *Curr Opin Infect Dis* 2000; 13:503–509.

5. Sartor RB. Pathogenesis and immune mechanisms of chronic inflammatory bowel diseases. *Am J Gastroenterol* 1997; 92:5S–11S.

6. Covacci AJ, Telford L, Del Giudice G, *et al.* *Helicobacter pylori* virulence and genetic geography. *Science* 1999; 284:1328–1333.

7. Blanchard TG, Czinn SJ, Nedrud JG. Host response and vaccine development to *Helicobacter pylori* infection. *Curr Top Microbiol Immunol* 1999; 241:181–213.

8. Finegold SM, Sutter VL. Fecal flora in different populations, with special reference to diet. *Am J Clin Nutr* 1978; 1:S116–S122.

9. Wilson KH, Blitchington RB. Human colonic biota studied by ribosomal DNA sequence analysis. *Appl Environ Microbiol* 1996; 62: 2273–2278.

10. Relman DA. The search for unrecognised pathogens. *Science* 1999; 284:1308–1311.

11. Walter J, Tannock GW, Tilsala-Timisjarvi A, *et al.* Detection and identification of gastrointestinal *Lactobacillus* species by using denaturing gradient gel electrophoresis and species-specific PCR primers. *Appl Environ Microbiol* 2000; 66:297–303.

12. Pahl A, Kuhlbrandt U, Brune K, *et al.* Quantitative detection of *Borrelia burgdorferi* by real-time PCR. *J Clin Microbiol* 1999; 37: 1958–1963.

13. Casten LA, Pierce SK. Receptor-mediated B cell antigen processing. Increased antigenicity of a globular protein covalently coupled to antibodies specific for B-cell surface structures. *J Immunol* 1988; 140:404–410.

14. Winter G, Griffiths AD, Hawkins RE, Hoogenboom HR. Making antibodies by phage display technology. *Annu Rev Immunol* 1994; 12:433–455.

15. Wei B, Dalwadi H, Gordon LK, *et al.* Molecular cloning of a *Bacteroides caccae* TonB-linked outer membrane protein inflammatory bowel disease identified by marker antibody. *Infect Immun* 2001; 69:6044–6054.

16. Siegel DL, Chang TY, Russell SL, Bunya VY. Isolation of cell surface-specific human monoclonal antibodies using phage display and magnetically-activated cell sorting: applications in immunohematology. *J Immunol Meth* 1997; 206:73–85.

17. Vaughn TJ, Williams AJ, Pritchard K, *et al.* Human antibodies with sub-nanomolar affinities isolated from a large non-immunised phage display library. *Nature Biotech* 1996; 14:309–314.

18. Cohavy O, Harth G, Horwitz MA, *et al.* Identification of a novel mycobacterial histone H1 homologue (HupB) as an antigenic target of pANCA monoclonal antibody and serum IgA from patients with Crohn's disease. *Infect Immun* 1999; 67:6510–6517.

19. Cohavy O, Bruckner D, Eggena ME, *et al.* Colonic bacteria express an ulcerative colitis pANCA-related protein epitope. *Infect Immun* 2000; 68:1542–1548.

20. Eggena M, Cohavy O, Parseghian M, *et al.* Identification of histone H1 as a cognate antigen of the ulcerative colitis-associated marker antibody pANCA. *J Autoimmun* 2000; 14:83–97.

21. Felgner PL, Liang X. Debugging expression screening. *Nature Biotechnol* 1999; 17: 329–330.

22. Emili AQ, Cagney G. Large-scale functional analysis using peptide or protein arrays. *Nature Biotech* 2000; 18:393–397.

23. Dalwadi H, Wei B, Braun J. Defining new pathogens and non-culturable infectious agents: the case of inflammatory bowel disease. *Curr Opin Gastroenterol* 2000; 16: 56–59.

24. Wei B, Huang T, Dalwadi H, *et al.* A Crohn's disease associated microbial gene and T-cell superantigen is a species-specific product of *Pseudomonas fluorescens. J Clin Invest* 2001 (submitted).

25. Sutton CL, Kim J, Yamane A, *et al.* Identification of a novel bacterial sequence associated with Crohn's disease. *Gastroenterology* 2000; 119:23–28.

26. Dalwadi H, Kronenberg M, Sutton CL, Braun J. The Crohn's disease-associated bacterial protein I2 is a novel enteric T cell superantigen. *Immun* 2001; 15:149–158.

The 'unculturables'

Kevin Collins and Liam O'Mahony

4

The flora of the gastrointestinal tract

Oesophagus

The human gastrointestinal tract is a complex and varied environment for microorganisms. Its beginning, the oesophagus, is a neuromuscular tube with a squamous epithelium. In real terms the oesophagus does not have a colonising commensal flora, but it may have transient bacterial flora from the oral cavity and from dietary sources. In certain circumstances human papilloma virus may also be found using DNA analysis with papilloma virus-specific probes. In immunocompromised patients (e.g. HIV/AIDS in SCID (severe combined immunodeficiency) patients and DiGeorge syndrome) the fungus *Candida albicans* may be present in high numbers. *C. albicans* may also be readily isolated from resected specimens from squamous carcinoma of the oesophagus.

Stomach

The stomach contents appear to have low levels of bacteria, in particular acid resistant lactobacilli. However, since the discovery of *Helicobacter pylori* by Warren and Marshall in 1983,[1] there has been a plethora of studies describing this hitherto unculturable micro-organism. These studies have been comprehensively reviewed elsewhere.[2]

The small intestine

In the upper small intestine, bile salts and pancreatic secretions destroy many orally acquired microorganisms. In addition, peristalsis maintains very low numbers at these sites. We have little if any information on unculturable flora from these sites. It is interesting to note that within hours of death, when peristalsis has ceased, the microbial flora flourishes.

The large intestine

Upon traversing the terminal ileum and into the caecum the microbial flora increases in number and diversity. Ultimately, in the large intestine, the numbers reach $\sim 10^{12}$ bacteria/gram of luminal contents. It is estimated that bacteria constitute one-third of the dry weight of faeces. The average person excretes between 10^{11} and 10^{14} bacteria in their faeces every day.

The 'unculturables'

In defining the microbial flora of the human gastrointestinal tract a major deficiency immediately becomes apparent: there are substantially more cells present than are measured using viable colony-forming units. In other words, the total number of bacteria that can be cultured is in the order of 10–20%. The remaining 80–90% are defined as unculturable. This is not altogether surprising when we consider that less than 1% of the microorganisms in nature have been cultured in the laboratory. Table 4.1 illustrates a number of questions frequently asked regarding the microbial flora. This list becomes more intriguing when we consider how little we know about the unculturables. However, we do know that normal full-term infants are born with a sterile meconium. Babies born with a blockage in the GI tract will have flora above the blockage but not below, indicating that bowel flora, both culturable and unculturable, are acquired through the oral cavity. A number of factors underpin our current inability to culture >80% of the human gastrointestinal flora (Table 4.2). The term 'unculturable' is really a functional definition which may be refined with time.

Recently developed molecular technologies can detect and semiquantify global flora (i.e. culturable and unculturable) without a prerequisite for cultivation. These methods are listed in Table 4.3. These technologies have brought about a renaissance in the analysis of the human intestinal flora. Before discussing selected techniques it is important to ask

Table 4.1
The potential benefits arising from accurate identification of the human gastrointestinal flora

- Acquisition of the gut flora
- Role in health and disease
- Influence of ageing
- Influence of diet
- Influence of antibiotics
- Influence of probiotics
- Influence of synbiotics

Table 4.2
The reasons underlying our inability to culture the majority of microbes present within the human gastrointestinal tract

- Dead cells
- Viable but unculturable – stressed cells
- Obligate requirements for coexisting flora
- Obligate requirements for host interactions or host-derived products
- Lack of knowledge regarding essential nutrients or culture conditions

Table 4.3
Molecular techniques currently being employed in the identification of the gastrointestinal flora

Molecular technologies	
PCR-based	DGGE/TGGE
	SSCP
	TRFLP
Probe-based	Dot blot
	FISH
	FISH Flow
	DNA Microarray
	DNA Microarray and
	MALDI-TOF-MS

Table 4.4
The faecal flora may not be representative of specific niche sites. Examples of such sites are illustrated

- Gastric flora
- Small bowel flora
- Ascending versus descending colon
- Luminal versus adherent flora
- Inflamed regions versus non-inflamed regions

questions about the material to be analysed. Most analysis, for obvious reasons of access and convenience, is performed on faeces. Table 4.4 illustrates a number of scenarios whereby faecal analysis may not be representative of niche sites. We need to analyse flora from many individuals of differing ethnicity, geography, age, life style, sex, etc. In addition, we need to examine the flora at different anatomical locations. For example, it has been estimated that in the large bowel the ratio of obligate anaerobes to facultative aerobes is 10,000:1, whereas the ratio in the crypts/mucosal surface is 10:1 (P. Borriello, personal communication). Therefore, even within a single organ there are specific environments within which different bacterial species thrive.

Molecular technologies

The introduction of 16S rRNA/DNA typing is rapidly gaining an important place in molecular microbial analysis of the human GI tract. Ribosomal RNA sequence analysis has many attractive features. First, rRNA is ubiquitous and highly conserved, yet also contains a number of variable regions in all prokaryotes, even in those yet to be discovered/identified. There is also an ever-increasing database of 16S RNA sequences. Figure 4.1 illustrates the structure of a ribosomal RNA operon from *Escherichia coli*.[3] As can be seen, the 16S rRNA operon has highly conserved sequences along with variable regions 1–9. Because rRNA is absolutely essential to the proper functioning of all organisms there is little divergence over evolutionary time. However, changes in the variable region (mutation rate) reflect evolutionary divergence and are species

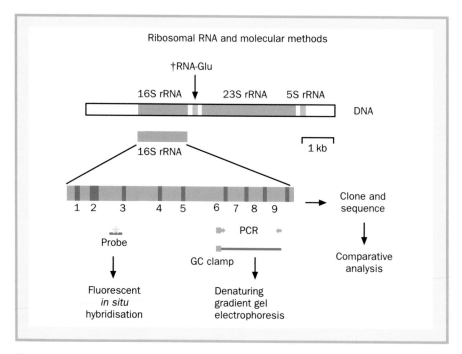

Figure 4.1
The structure of a ribosomal 16S RNA operon.

specific. Cloning and sequencing of 16rRNA genes is therefore an attractive method of phylogenetic classification for microorganisms.

To analyse dominant organisms (both culturable and unculturable) rapidly, in complex communities, the 16rRNA genes have been analysed using polymerase chain reaction (PCR) with universal 16S RNA primers spanning conserved and variable regions. Incorporated in one of the primers is a GC-rich clamp to prevent complete dissociation of the strands under a strong denaturing chemical gradient or an increasing temperature gradient. In practice, total microbial DNA is extracted from faecal samples (using glass or zirconium beads). DNA is extracted from all microbial species in the specimen. Using primers and PCR as outlined, 16S rDNA (also RT-PCR 16S rRNA)[4] can be amplified. In theory, the more dominant the organism, the more intense the specific PCR product. Denaturing gradient gel electrophoresis (DGGE) is used to separate the individual PCR products. Figure 4.2

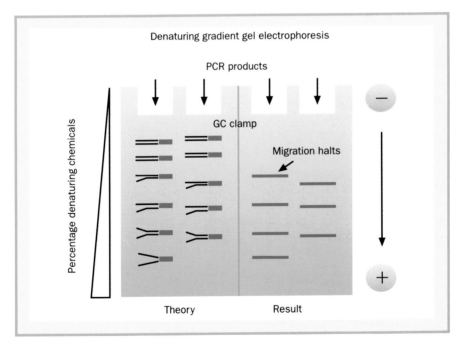

Figure 4.2
Schematic representation of the principles underlying DGGE.

illustrates the concept of DGGE. The complex mixture of PCR products is electrophoresed through a polyacrylamide gel containing an increasing gradient of denaturing chemicals (usually urea and formamide). The double-stranded PCR products will have variable sequences and therefore different melting points. Once a specific melting point is reached, dissociation occurs, except at the GC clamp. The open pinlike structure slows dramatically or stops migrating in the gel. This gives rise to a specific band. In practice, bands can be separated based on a single nucleotide difference. Following staining of the gel, a banding pattern can be observed which reflects the diversity of the rRNA genes in the sample. Human adult faecal samples usually yield approximately 20 dominant bands representing, on a semiquantitative basis, the most abundant species within the faecal flora. Temperature gradient gel electrophoresis (TGGE) uses the same principle except that the chemical denaturing gradient is replaced by an increasing temperature denaturing gradient. An example of such a profile can be seen in Figure 4.3. These are data generated using one sample from a probiotic feeding study[5] whereby a probiotic lactobacillus UCC 118 was fed to healthy adults at 10^{10} viable cells per day for 3 weeks. A control group consumed a placebo product once a day for 3 weeks. Faecal samples were taken at time 0 and after 3 weeks. They were analysed using

conventional culture techniques for total lactobacilli counts, bacteroides, bifidobacteria and coliforms. Samples were also analysed by DGGE.[3]

Using standard microbiological culture techniques at week 0, a considerable range in the numbers of each bacterial species was seen between different individuals (e.g. 1000-fold difference in lactobacilli, 10^6–10^9/g). After probiotic feeding significant changes were seen in the test group only (all subjects achieved $\geq$ 10^8 lactobacilli/g). From Figure 4.3 it can be seen that DGGE analysis confirms that there is a great diversity in flora between individuals. However, it demonstrated that probiotic feeding had little discernible effect

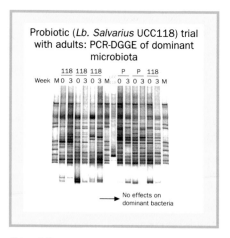

Probiotic (*Lb. Salvarius* UCC118) trial with adults: PCR-DGGE of dominant microbiota

No effects on dominant bacteria

Figure 4.3
DGGE was performed on faecal samples isolated pre and postprobiotic (118) or placebo (P) consumption. No substantial differences were noted.

on the dominant flora as detected using DGGE.

Individual bands from DGGE/TGGE gels can be excised and sequenced, thereby potentially identifying the bacterial strain without cultivation steps. Coupling this to the ever-increasing 16S rRNA databank, it is anticipated that the use of DGGE in global dominant flora analysis under such influences of antibiotics, probiotics, prebiotics, disease, etc. will increase. These techniques can be refined using primers which are genus specific, species specific and even strain specific, e.g. to track a specific probiotic strain. In addition, hybridisation probes can be synthesised and used to identify DGGE/TGGE bands on a genus, species and even strain basis.

Other techniques currently in use are single-strand conformation polymorphism (SSCP)[6] and terminal restriction fragment length polymorphism (TRFLP).[7] Although the widespread application of PCR techniques in the analysis of human gastrointestinal flora is awaited with great expectation, some word of caution must be expressed. Extraction of DNA/RNA from all cells must be achieved efficiently and equally. Using current methodologies this is most unlikely. There are also potential problems with fidelity of the polymerase enzyme in the PCR reactions: there may be increasing numbers of mutations, chimeras and heteroduplexes formed with increasing PCR cycle numbers.[8] In addition, primers may preferentially amplify certain species in such a diverse environment. Furthermore, there may be heterogeneity in multicopy 16S rDNA genes for any given strain, e.g. *Bifidobacterium adolentis.*[9]

Probe-based technologies

With an ever-increasing amount of sequence data becoming available for both unculturable and culturable gut microbes, substantial efforts have focused on generating ribosomal RNA-based hybridisation probes for studying the complex ecology of human gut flora. These probes, incorporating molecular beacons that fluoresce following hybridisation,[10] are currently being used for fluorescent *in-situ* hybridisation analysis (FISH) using fluorescent or confocal laser scanning microscopy. A further advance on this technique is the ability to combine FISH with flow cytometry. Flow FISH has the advantage of counting each cell as a single event and at least four different probes can be used simultaneously on a single sample (four probes with four fluorochromes emitting light at different wavelengths). In addition, it can be automated and large amounts of data can be captured for subsequent analysis.

DNA microarray or DNA chip technology is another promising technique for the identification and characterisation of the gastrointestinal microflora. Again, with increasing genomics information the gene array chip can incorporate thousands of designer probes for genus, species and strain identification. This reaction is typically fluorescence based. Light emitted from the chip is electronically recorded and the data are captured for subsequent multiparametric analysis. Gene array technology could potentially evaluate microbial activity, e.g. ribosomal RNA content (the higher the ribosome count the more metabolically active the organism). The expression of specific mRNA sequences could be examined. Finally, the combination of DNA microarrays and sequencing by hybridisation using MALDI-TOF-MS (matrix-assisted laser desorption ionisation time of flight mass spectrometry) is becoming a reality.[11]

Discussion

Using the techniques outlined above we may ultimately answer the questions that William de Vos proposes regarding the gastrointestinal flora, i.e.:

- Who is in there?
- How many of you are there?
- Who are you talking to?
- What are you doing?
- Do I like it?
- If not, what do I do?

The use of these techniques will allow us to gain access to hitherto untapped sources of microbial genomes. We will then progress

into proteomics in order to answer the questions as to what these organisms are doing and whether we like it or not, e.g. the production of desirable metabolites such as vitamins or toxins/carcinogens.

Acknowledgements

We would like to thank Elaine Vaughan, William de Vos and Anton Ackermans for their assistance in preparing this article.

References

1. Warren JR, Marshall BJ. Unidentified curved bacilli: on gastric mucosa epithelium in active gastritis. *Lancet* 1983; I:1273.

2. Farthing MJG. *Helicobacter pylori* infection: an overview. *Br Med Bull* 1998; 554:1–6.

3. Vaughan EE, Heilig HG, Zoetendal EG, *et al.* Molecular approaches to study probiotic bacteria. *Trends Food Sci Tech* 1999; 10: 400–404.

4. Zoetendal EG, Akkermans ADL, de Vos WM. Temperature gradient gel electrophoresis analysis of 16S rRNA from human fecal samples reveals stable and host-specific communities of active bacteria. *Appl Environ Microbiol* 1998; 64:3854–3859.

5. Dunne C, Murphy L, Flynn S, *et al.* Probiotics: from myth to reality. Demonstration of functionality in animal models of disease and in human clinical trials. *Antoine Van Leeuwenhoek* 1999; 76:279–292.

6. Schwieger F, Tebbe CC. A new approach to utilise PCR-single-strand-conformation polymorphism for 16S rRNA gene-based

microbial community analysis. *Appl Environ Microbiol* 1998; 64:4870–4876.

7. Marsh TL. Terminal restriction fragment length polymorphism (T-RFLP): an emerging method for characterising diversity among homologous populations of amplification products. *Curr Opin Microbiol* 1999; 2: 323–327.

8. Qiu X, Wu L, Huang H, *et al.* Evaluation of PCR-generated chimeras, mutations, and heteroduplexes with 16S rRNA gene based cloning. *Appl Environ Microbiol* 2001; 67:880–887.

9. Satokari RM, Vaughan EE, Akkermans ADL, *et al.* Bifidobacterial diversity in human feces detected by genus-specific PCR and denaturing gel electrophoresis. *Appl Environ Microbiol* 2001; 67:504–513.

10. Tyagi S, Kramer FR. Molecular beacons: probes that fluoresce upon hybridisation. *Nature Biotech* 1996; 14:303–307.

11. Eickhoff H, Ivanov I, Kietzmann M, *et al.* Robotic equipment and microsystem technology in biological research. In: Kohler JM, Mejevaia T, Saluz HP, eds. *Microsystem Technology: a powerful tool for biomolecular studies.* Basel: Birkhauser Verlag, *BioMethods* 1999; 10:17–30.

Summary and observations

Per Falk and Tore Midtvedt

Reading this section probably takes us back to our school days. The previous four chapters have presented the most complex ecosystem, consisting of microbial and host cells. In all multicellular organisms the tube from mouth to anus represents an exciting playground for simple, as well as elaborate, microbe–microbe and microbe–host interactions. The number of microbes is overwhelming, both in terms of total numbers and in component species. In addition, the metabolic capacity of the microflora is impressive and can have a fundamental impact on the host. The fact that there are more bacteria in one gram of human large bowel contents than there have ever been humans on the planet is an excellent illustration of this. While we are on the subject of gut microflora trivia, it has been calculated that one *Escherichia coli* could multiply to a mass greater than our planet in less than two days, if it could be kept in a constant log-phase with free access to nutrition.

A simple question has to be asked: Do we know enough to describe the impact of the gut microflora on human physiology? As stated by the first author: 'the microbial ecology of the gut is still very poorly understood, in terms of both composition and function, and factors that may alter the flora'. Taking a historical view, we can comment that species such as *Clostridium difficile, Campylobacter jejuni* and *Helicobacter pylori,* were all relatively recently identified and recognised as main players in the gastrointestinal ecosystem. Naturally, they have been transient or persistent colonisers of our gastrointestinal tract for much longer, and it goes without saying that many more unknown components of the gut ecosystem with a significant impact on physiology and pathology will be identified, as we now can apply tools with con-siderably higher resolution than ever before.

Another simple question has to be asked: Why, then, are we just at the end of the beginning and not at the beginning of the end? The answer(s) was (were) given by the authors:

- Difficulties in obtaining adequate samples from several sites within the GI tract;
- Methodological limitations;
- An underestimation of the complexity of the system.

As outlined by one of the authors, 'obtaining specimens from any site other than the mouth and anus in healthy volunteers is difficult'. In patients, invasive techniques such as gastroscopy and colonoscopy can be used to harvest materials from both ends of the GI tract. However, the major part of the small intestine remains beyond reach. From a bacteriological point of view this important part of the gut still represents a *terra incognita*. For obvious reasons, collection of materials from operations, often in emergency situations involving trauma, does not solve the problem of obtaining adequate samples.

As mentioned by Tannock, 'much of our knowledge of the composition of the gut microflora of humans is derived from bacteriological studies that utilised the traditional techniques of culture, microscopy and the determination of the fermentative and other biochemical capabilities of bacterial isolates'. Over the years there have been several methodological improvements, for instance anaerobic glove boxes, test tubes flushed with an oxygen-free gas, etc., but we still do have to 'admit that the success of phenotypic identification methods often relies on the experience of the laboratory worker and a dose of intuition'.

The contributions from Tannock, Braun and Collins clearly indicate that a new era is emerging. It is easy to forecast that the application of molecular methods will dramatically increase our knowledge about the composition of the flora. We will be able to recognise 'the unculturables', to pinpoint more biologically significant species, and to follow age-, genetic-, environment-, and disease-related variations and differences in the flora. However, the data should be interpreted with great caution. The authors have given us several examples of the problems in generalising based on too-small groups or cohorts.

A provocative question has to be asked: So what? We should realise that the presence in faeces of genetic material from microbe X or Y provides no indication as to the role of these microbes in their natural niche, often located elsewhere in the GI tract. In other words, improvements in our knowledge about the composition of the flora have to be linked to a deeper understanding about flora-related functions and interactions. Therefore, the future is not 'no culture, just genotype'. The future is a combination of new and old methods in order to understand the molecular correlates to the host–microbial cross-talk that is continuously ongoing – from cradle to grave, and in health and disease. That is *the* major challenge, for the scientific community as well as for the pharmaceutical companies.

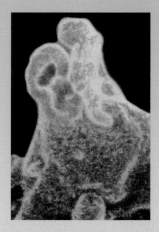

PART 2

The host response to the normal intestinal flora

Immune regulation of the normal intestinal bacterial flora

Andrew J Macpherson, Therese Uhr and Alain Lamarre

5

Introduction

Despite the immense density of bacteria in the lower intestine of mammals it is relatively unusual for intestinal or systemic problems to occur, at least when man is healthy and has good hygiene conditions in the developed world, or when immunocompetent experimental animals are housed in a pathogen-free facility. This is hardly surprising, since vertebrates have coevolved with their commensal intestinal bacterial flora, and so they are adept at confining most of the flora to the intestinal lumen and highly efficient at clearing those bacteria that penetrate the physical and immune defences. In this chapter we will describe the nature of mucosal immune defences against commensal organisms, and the immune consequences when bacteria penetrate to systemic secondary lymphoid tissues, including the spleen and peripheral lymph nodes.

Bacteria from the commensal intestinal flora can penetrate into the body and reach extraintestinal sites

Whereas normal individuals rarely have problems from their intestinal flora, in immunosuppressed patients these can cause serious infections, especially in those undergoing chemotherapy or bone marrow transplantation, or in patients with end-stage AIDS.[1,2] Septicaemia from commensal organisms is also seen in elderly debilitated patients. This appears to be the tip of an iceberg, because commensal organisms can frequently be cultured from the mesenteric lymph nodes even in patients without obvious mucosal intestinal disease.[3]

The penetration of commensal intestinal bacteria into underlying tissues is defined as 'translocation'. This has been studied in experimental animals, where commensal organisms are not cultured from mesenteric lymph nodes or other systemic tissues of 'wild-type' immunocompetent animals, but are spontaneously translocated to the mesenteric lymph nodes, spleen, liver and kidneys in T-cell-deficient athymic (nude) mice.[4] Such translocation also occurs in animals depleted of CD4 or CD8 T cells.[5,6] The consequences of translocation are not severe if the bactericidal mechanisms of phagocytes are unimpaired – whereas they are fatal in mice that are deficient for key microbiocidal enzymes within phagocytes as a result of a combination of two targeted genetic lesions – phagocyte oxidase (which results in the production of oxygen free radicals) and the inducible form of nitric oxide (gp91[phox-/-]/NOS2[-/-]).[7] Cells from these gp91[phox-/-]/NOS2[-/-] mice cannot kill phagocytosed microorganisms, and they succumb to sepsis from commensal bacteria by the age of 4 weeks (on the C57BL/6 background), despite the use of pathogen-free conditions and prophylactic antibiotics. Because gp91[phox-/-]/NOS2[-/-] mice are otherwise immunocompetent, it follows that even with intact adaptive immunity there can be very low levels of commensal bacterial penetration, which are sufficient to cause fatal sepsis if the penetrating bacteria cannot be killed after phagocytosis.

The immune system of a clean immunocompetent animal is systemically ignorant, but not tolerant, of its intestinal flora

When mice are kept in specific pathogen-free (SPF) conditions the systemic immune system is ignorant of the commensal flora. This was shown by looking at priming reactions for IgG specific for commensal bacterial proteins in the serum of SPF C57BL/6 wild-type mice.[8] Whereas the unmanipulated animals have no specific IgG in the serum, they are not 'tolerant' because an intravenous injection of as few as 10^6 cfu (colony-forming units) of a dominant aerobic commensal bacterium (which is present at 10^{7-9} cfu/g of lower intestinal contents) will reproducibly induce IgG responses against the bacterial cell wall proteins.

Although young immunocompetent animals kept free of pathogens do not have significant levels of commensal bacterial translocation, adult humans do have evidence of systemic priming of serum IgG to intestinal bacteria,[9] so presumably translocation of commensal bacteria does occur in the real world, where intestinal infections, or other insults to the permeability barrier of the epithelial cell layer, periodically facilitate the penetration of organisms that are within the intestinal lumen.

Possible consequences on systemic immunity of translocation of commensal bacteria

Does penetration of commensal bacteria matter? Since it is clear that innate immune mechanisms (which do not require an immunological learning effect of prior exposure to antigen for their effectiveness) can eliminate the flora that penetrate the physical and immune mucosal immune defences, what are the consequences of bacterial translocation for the systemic immune system?

In this section we principally discuss the consequences of translocation on systemic immunity, although it is clear from both animal models and studies of human disease that bacterial products derived from the commensal intestinal flora can induce local inflammatory reactions within the intestinal mucosa itself. This results in spontaneous intestinal inflammation in a wide variety of

genetically targeted and immune manipulated animal models (reviewed in reference 10), and inflammatory bowel disease in human individuals that are genetically predisposed.[11–13]

A comparison of immunoglobulin- and antibody-producing cell levels in germ-free and conventional animals shows dramatic increases, especially of the IgG, IgA and IgE isotypes, when bacteria are present in the intestine.[14–17] Overall levels of mucosal and systemic antibodies are therefore critically dependent on the presence of the intestinal flora. This leads to the question of whether the flora also influences the primary repertoire – that is, the constellation of binding specificities that exist before the immune system is challenged by a pathogen.

Antibodies are produced following a process of somatic recombination of the DNA encoding the light and heavy chains in the developing B cell, when one of each of the multiple V (D)$_{heavy\ chain}$ and J gene segments are recombined to form a unit that can be transcribed with the constant region. The selection of V, D and J segments is not random, and some are overrepresented in the preimmune (naïve) repertoire.[18] Later this primary repertoire is diversified during immune reactions, when the affinity of antibody binding is optimised by mutations particularly at the coding regions for the critical sites of antigen–antibody contact, and possibly by a process of receptor revision which swaps suboptimal V gene segments in immature B cells that still express RAG genes.[19–21] Experiments on mice that initially have a monoclonal repertoire because of genetic targeting of a defined VDJ segment into the correct genetic position upstream of μ heavy chain locus certainly diversify from this specificity (nitrophenyl) with increasing age, and the pattern of V segment usage suggests that this may be an effect of the intestinal bacteria.[22,23] It has also been shown that the accumulation of somatic mutations in serum immunoglobulins is dependent on exposure to environmental antigens,[24] of which the commensal flora are likely to be the predominant influence. This means that the preimmune primary B-cell repertoire may be dramatically influenced by the intestinal flora, although whether live commensal bacterial translocation is required for this process, and the site(s) where diversification occurs (mesenteric lymph nodes, spleen, extrasplenic non-mesenteric secondary lymphoid tissues) remain unclear.

It can be argued that the primary immune repertoire has been derived from coevolution of mammals with their pathogens,[25–27] so there may be a delicate balance between diversification mechanisms in response to what are essentially superfluous systemic anticommensal immune responses and preservation of the primary repertoire. Clearly, the survival of an animal or human following exposure to a novel infection depends on the quality of the primary immune response, and in some infectious models premature diversification makes the animal particularly susceptible.[28]

Studies of T-cell receptor gene usage indicate that the presence of the flora makes much less difference to the primary repertoire of T-cell subsets,[29–31] which can be rationalised by the fact that positive and negative selection of the preimmune repertoire of most systemic T cells takes place in the sterile environment of the thymus in response to low or high affinities of the T-cell receptor of each developing cell to self antigens. There are certainly later selection and deletional events in response to environmental antigens, for example during induction of oral tolerance[32] – but the effects on the preimmune T-cell repertoire are probably small compared with those on the B-cell repertoire.

Immune adaptation of animals to their commensal bacterial flora

Although innate immune mechanisms are essential for the successful handling of the commensal bacteria, the flora has enormous effects on the composition and functioning of the adaptive components of the mucosal immune system. This was initially apparent from examining germ-free animals which are born and maintained in a completely sterile environment (so they have no intestinal bacteria whatsoever). When compared with animals of the same strain maintained under conventional or specific pathogen-free husbandry conditions, the germ-free animals have tiny Peyer's patches, very low contents of IgA-producing cells in the mucosa, and reduced contents of CD8αβ cells and CD4+ cells in the intraepithelial and lamina propria respectively.[16,17,33] Cebra and his colleagues have studied the events that occur following the introduction of a single bacterial species (*Morganella morganii*) from the commensal flora in mice that were initially germ-free and were maintained in an environment that was sterile (apart from the *Morganella*) throughout the experiment.[34] Initially the production of intestinal IgA was very low, and the colonising bacteria were not successfully confined to the intestinal lumen, but could be cultured from the mesenteric lymph nodes and the spleen for up to 100 days. The reduction of this bacterial translocation coincided with induction of the intestinal IgA response; although this does not mean that IgA necessarily limits the exposure of the mucosa and underlying tissues to the commensal bacteria, because other immune and structural changes occur as the germ-free intestine is colonised by bacteria. The experiments do show that adaptation by the intestine and mucosal immune system is important in limiting the exposure of body tissues to a defined commensal intestinal organism.

A special case of adaptative immune responses to the commensal flora may exist in the antibodies of maternal milk. Cebra's laboratory has also shown that when immunocompetent (*scid/+*) neonatal mice receive milk from an immunoincompetent (*scid/scid*) mother, activation of the mucosal immune system occurs before weaning, whereas this is delayed until the time of weaning when the mother is immunocompetent (*scid/+*).[35] These experiments look at the effects of adaptive immune lactational responses (including postnatal IgG uptake through the milk), but not innate factors, because these are present in milk of both *scid/+* and *scid/scid* dams.

The neonate is obviously especially susceptible to challenges from pathogens and environmental commensal organisms during the time that it takes for its own immune system to mature, and much of the commensal flora is rapidly acquired from other family members soon after birth.[36] IgA is the predominant immunoglobulin in milk, and the immune experience of the mother may allow secretion of IgA that is appropriate to prevalent mucosal pathogens and, more speculatively, it may limit the penetration of commensal bacteria across the immature neonatal intestine. Whereas early in lactation polymeric IgA is transported from the serum across mammary epithelia, later there are local IgA-producing plasma cells within the mammary gland (including those that have been induced in maternal intestinal lymphoid tissues).[35,37–39]

Mechanisms of induction of adaptive immune responses to the commensal intestinal bacterial flora

Classic experiments showed that induction of both IgA[+] B cells and some mucosal T cells in the intestine occurs in the Peyer's patches.[40–43] These cells recirculate through the intestinal lymph and via the mesenteric lymph nodes to enter the bloodstream at the level of the thoracic duct, and complete their journey through the blood back to the intestine (and to other mucosal sites). It is well established that the Peyer's patches are a site of adaptive mucosal responses.

More recently another source of intestinal T cells has been described: these are cryptopatches which consist of small collections of immature T cells deep to the epithelial layer of the crypt enterocytes.[44,45] They have been shown to be lymphopoietic sites for the TCRγδ and TCRαβ intraepithelial T cells, but these subsets are produced in germ-free animals, so whether there is an adaptive component to T-cell ontogeny in these structures remains unclear. They have *not* been shown to be a source of intestinal B cells.

Induction of IgA in the Peyer's patches has previously been thought to be a process that is highly dependent on T–B-cell interactions, largely from experiments with the oral adjuvant cholera toxin.[46, 47] However, despite the abolition of the cholera toxin response in strains of mice deficient in T cells or in the cytokine or signalling interactions required for T–B-cell interactions, these strains still contain significant IgA-secreting plasma cells within the intestinal lamina propria.[48–50] We have shown that the IgA content of the strain that is T-cell deficient as a result of two targeted lesions affecting the β and δ chains of the T-cell receptor (TCRβ[−/−] δ[−/−], affecting αβ T cells and γδ T cells, respectively) is about a quarter of that present in wild-type controls. Despite the absence of T-cell help in this strain, it can induce IgA responses to proteins and other cell wall components of commensal bacteria similar to those found in wild-type animals.[8] Thus, the IgA responses to commensal bacteria (unlike those to toxins) do not necessarily require help from T cells.

It is known that there are two potential sources of B cells in adult rodents – the bone marrow (giving rise to B2 cells) and the pleuroperitoneal cavity (B1 cells). The relatively undifferentiated forms of these B1 and B2 cells can be distinguished by their surface markers,[51–54] but the characteristic surface proteins are no longer expressed by the time either lineage has differentiated into plasma cells. To find out which of these gives rise to T-independent IgA, we made radiation chimeras in which $TCR\beta^{-/-} \delta^{-/-}$ animals were lethally irradiated to destroy the endogenous haematopoietic cells, and then reconstituted with bone marrow (including B2 cells) expressing the IgA^b allotype, and B1 cells expressing the IgA^a allotype.[8] Measurements of the relative contributions of IgA^a and IgA^b allotypes in the intestinal IgA of the reconstituted animal allowed us to show that most of the intestinal T-independent IgA was derived from B1 cells.

Many of the B cells in humans are CD5$^+$ (one of the surface markers associated with B1 cells), especially early life,[55,56] but attempts to determine whether it contributes to human intestinal IgA have necessarily been made indirectly by looking at B2-associated mutations in DNA or RNA from IgA plasma cells.[57–59] This approach has largely been applied to adults, and the sequence comparisons have been with database information from unrelated individuals, so the relative contribution of the B1 lineage to human intestinal IgA remains uncertain.

IgA with specificities against the commensal intestinal flora is much more effectively induced in the intestine than in the serum, so there appears to be some separation in the mucosal and systemic IgA.[8] Indeed, it is possible to show that serum IgA can be induced quite independently of intestinal lymphoid tissues in alymphoplastic (aly/aly) mice (which lack Peyer's patches and secondary lymphoid structures other than the spleen) following irradiation and reconstitution with wild-type bone marrow.[60] Thus intestinal IgA responses to the commensal flora are functionally and mechanistically distinct from serum responses.

Function of adaptive responses in protecting against penetration of the commensal bacteria

Whereas it is clear that the intestine undergoes substantial changes in adapting to the presence of the commensal intestinal flora, the alterations in cellular metabolism and makeup of the mucosa play an important part in this, so the precise contributions of innate and adaptive immunity in this process have yet to be defined. There is some evidence in T-cell-deficient mice that commensal translocation is increased,[6] and in mice with a targeted deletion of IgA there is increased systemic priming of anticommensal IgG reactions,[8] so adaptive responses of both arms of the mucosal immune system probably contribute to the protective function. The details of mucosal immune mechanisms that limit systemic exposure to commensals, and the functional consequences over time of such exposure in immunocompetent animals, remain to be determined.

Acknowledgements

The authors wish to thank Professors Rolf Zinkernagel and Hans Hengartner for their encouragement and support.

References

1. Tancrede CH, Andremont AO. Bacterial translocation and gram-negative bacteremia in patients with hematological malignancies. *J Infect Dis* 1985; 152:99–103.

2. Witt DJ, Craven DE, McCabe WR. Bacterial infections in adult patients with the acquired immune deficiency syndrome (AIDS) and AIDS-related complex. *Am J Med* 1987; 82: 900–906.

3. O'Boyle CJ, MacFie J, Mitchell CJ, *et al.* Microbiology of bacterial translocation in humans. *Gut* 1998; 42:29–35.

4. Owens WE, Berg RD. Bacterial translocation from the gastrointestinal tract of athymic (nu/nu) mice. *Infect Immun* 1980; 27: 461–467.

5. Berg RD. The indigenous gastrointestinal microflora. *Trends Microbiol* 1996; 4: 430–435.

6. Gautreaux MD, Gelder FB, Deitch EA, Berg RD. Adoptive transfer of T lymphocytes to T-cell-depleted mice inhibits *Escherichia coli* translocation from the gastrointestinal tract. *Infect Immun* 1995; 63:3827–3834.

7. Shiloh MU, MacMicking JD, Nicholson S, *et al.* Phenotype of mice and macrophages deficient in both phagocyte oxidase and inducible nitric oxide synthase. *Immunity* 1999; 10:29–38.

8. Macpherson AJ, Gatto D, Sainsbury E, *et al.* A primitive T cell-independent mechanism of intestinal mucosal IgA responses to commensal bacteria. *Science* 2000; 288: 2222–2226.

9. Macpherson AJ, Khoo UY, Forgacs I, Philpott-Howard J, Bjarnason I. Mucosal antibodies in inflammatory bowel disease are directed against intestinal bacteria. *Gut* 1996; 38:365–375.

10. Simpson SJ, de Jong YP, Comiskey M, Terhorst C. T cells in mouse models of gut inflammation. *Chem Immunol* 1998; 71: 118–138.

11. Ogura Y, Bonen DK, Inohara N, *et al.* A frameshift mutation in NOD2 associated with susceptibility to Crohn's disease. *Nature* 2001; 411:603–606.

12. Hugot JP, Chamaillard M, Zouali H, *et al.* Association of NOD2 leucine-rich repeat variants with susceptibility to Crohn's disease. *Nature* 2001; 411:599–603.

13. Hampe J, Cuthbert A, Croucher PJP, *et al.* Association between insertion mutation in NOD2 gene and Crohn's disease in German and British populations. *Lancet* 2001; 357: 1925–1928.

14. Haury M, Sundblad A, Grandien A, *et al.* The repertoire of IgM in normal mice is largely independent of external antigenis contact. *Eur J Immunol* 1997; 27:1557–1563.

15. Hooijkaas H, Benner R, Pleasants JR, Wostmann BS. Isotypes and specificities of immunoglobulins produced by germ-free mice fed chemically defined ultrafiltered 'antigen-free' diet. *Eur J Immunol* 1984; 14:1127–1130.

16. Schaedler RW, Dubos R, Costello R. Association of germfree mice with bacteria

isolated from normal mice. *J Exp Med* 1965;
122:77–83.

17. Moreau MC, Ducluzeau R, Guy-Grand D,
Muller MC. Increase in the population of
duodenal immunoglobulin A plasmocytes in
axenic mice associated with different living or
dead bacterial strains of intestinal origin.
Infect Immun 1978; 21:532–539.

18. Kearney JF, Won WJ, Benedict C, *et al.* B cell
development in mice. *Int Rev Immunol* 1997;
15:207–241.

19. Tonegawa S. Somatic generation of antibody
diversity. *Nature* 1983; 302:575–581.

20. Perlmutter RM, Kearney JF, Chang SP, Hood
LE. Developmentally controlled expression of
immunoglobulin VH genes. *Science* 1985;
227:1597–1601.

21. Monroe RJ, Seidl KJ, Gaertner F, *et al.*
RAG2:GFP knockin mice reveal novel aspects
of RAG2 expression in primary and peripheral
lymphoid tissues. *Immunity* 1999; 11:
201–212.

22. Cascalho M, Ma A, Lee S, Masat L, Wabl M.
A quasi-monoclonal mouse. *Science* 1996;
272:1649–1652.

23. Cascalho M, Wong J, Wabl M. VH gene
replacement in hyperselected B cells of the
quasimonoclonal mouse. *J Immunol* 1997;
159:5795–5801.

24. Williams GT, Jolly CJ, Kohler J, Neuberger
MS. The contribution of somatic
hypermutation to the diversity of serum
immunoglobulin: dramatic increase with age.
Immunity 2000; 13:409–417.

25. Briles DE, Nahem M, Schroer K, *et al.*
Antiphosphocholine antibodies found in
normal mouse serum are protective against
intravenous infection with type 3

Streptococcus pneumoniae. J Exp Med 1981;
153:694.

26. Ochsenbein AF, Fehr T, Lutz C, *et al.*
Control of early viral and bacterial
distribution and disease by natural antibodies.
Science 1999; 286:2156–2159.

27. Zinkernagel RM. On immunological
memory. *Phil Trans Roy Soc Lond B Biol Sci*
2000; 355:369–371.

28. Benedict CL, Kearney JF. Increased junctional
diversity in fetal B cells results in a loss of
protective anti-phosphorylcholine antibodies
in adult mice. *Immunity* 1999; 10:607–617.

29. Vos Q, Jones LA, Kruisbeek AM. Mice
deprived of exogenous antigenic stimulation
develop a normal repertoire of functional T
cells. *J Immunol* 1992; 149:1204–1210.

30. Bousso P, Lemaitre F, Laouini D,
Kanellopoulos J, Kourilsky P. The peripheral
CD8 T cell repertoire is largely independent
of the presence of intestinal flora. *Int
Immunol* 2000; 12:425–430.

31. Park SH, Guy-Grand D, Lemonnier FA, *et al.*
Selection and expansion of CD8alpha/alpha T
cell receptor alpha/beta intestinal
intraepithelial lymphocytes in the absence of
both classical major histocompatibility
complex class I and nonclassical CD1
molecules. *J Exp Med* 1999; 190:885–890.

32. Gutgemann I, Fahrer AM, Altman JD, Davis
MM, Chien YH. Induction of rapid T cell
activation and tolerance by systemic
presentation of an orally administered antigen.
Immunity 1998; 8:667–673.

33. Helgeland L, Vaage JT, Rolstad B, Midtvedt
T, Brandtzaeg P. Microbial colonization
influences composition and T-cell receptor V
beta repertoire of intraepithelial lymphocytes

in rat intestine. *Immunology* 1996; 89: 494–501.

34. Shroff KE, Meslin K, Cebra JJ. Commensal enteric bacteria engender a self-limiting humoral mucosal immune response while permanently colonizing the gut. *Infect Immun* 1995; 63:3904–3913.

35. Kramer DR, Cebra JJ. Early appearance of 'natural' mucosal IgA responses and germinal centers in suckling mice developing in the absence of maternal antibodies. *J Immunol* 1995; 154:2051–2062.

36. Mackie R, Sghir A, Gaskins HR. Developmental microbial ecology of the neonatal gastrointestinal tract. *Am J Clin Nutr* 1999; 69:1035S–1045S.

37. Roux ME, McWilliams M, Phillips-Quagliata JM, Weisz-Carrington P, Lamm ME. Origin of IgA-secreting plasma cells in the mammary gland. *J Exp Med* 1977; 146:1311–1322.

38. Halsey JF, Mitchell C, Meyer R, Cebra JJ. Metabolism of immunoglobulin A in lactating mice: origins of immunoglobulin A in milk. *Eur J Immunol* 1982; 12:107–112.

39. Weisz-Carrington P, Roux ME, McWilliams M, JM P-Q, Lamm ME. Organ and isotype distribution of plasma cells producing specific antibody after oral immunization: evidence for a generalized secretory immune system. *J Immunol* 1979; 123:1705–8.

40. Craig SW, Cebra JJ. Peyer's patches: an enriched source of precursors for IgA-producing immunocytes in the rabbit. *J Exp Med* 1971; 134:188–200.

41. Husband AJ, Gowans JL. The origin and antigen-dependent distribution of IgA-containing cells in the intestine. *J Exp Med* 1978; 148:1146–1160.

42. Pierce NF, Gowans JL. Cellular kinetics of the

intestinal immune response to cholera toxoid in rats. *J Exp Med* 1975; 142:1550–1563.

43. Guy-Grand D, Griscelli C, Vassalli P. The gut-associated lymphoid system: nature and properties of the large dividing cells. *Eur J Immunol* 1974; 4:435–443.

44. Saito H, Kanamori Y, Takemori T, *et al.* Generation of intestinal T cells from progenitors residing in gut cryptopatches. *Science* 1998; 280:275–278.

45. Kanamori Y, Ishimaru K, Nanno M, *et al.* Identification of novel lymphoid tissues in murine intestinal mucosa where clusters of c-kit+ IL-7R+ Thy1+ lympho-hemopoietic progenitors develop. *J Exp Med* 1996; 184: 1449–1459.

46. Guy-Grand D, Griscelli C, Vassalli P. Peyer's patches, gut IgA plasma cells and thymic function: study in nude mice bearing thymic grafts. *J Immunol* 1975; 115:361–364.

47. Lycke N, Eriksen L, Holmgren J. Protection against cholera toxin after oral immunisation is thymus dependent and associated with intestinal production of neutralising IgA antitoxin. *Scand J Immunol* 1987; 25:413–419.

48. Hörnquist CE, Ekman L, Grdic KD, Schön K, Lycke NY. Paradoxical IgA immunity in CD4-deficient mice. *J Immunol* 1995; 155:2877–2887.

49. Vajdy M, Kosco-Vilbois MH, Kopf M, Kohler G, Lycke N. Impaired mucosal immune responses in interleukin 4-targeted mice. *J Exp Med* 1995; 181:41–53.

50. Gardby E, Lane P, Lycke NY. Requirements for B7-CD28 costimulation in mucosal IgA responses: paradoxes observed in CTLA4-H gamma 1 transgenic mice. *J Immunol* 1998; 161:49–59.

51. Melchers F, Rolink A. B-lymphocyte development and biology. In: Paul WE, ed. *Fundamental Immunology* 4th edn. Philadelphia: Lippincott-Raven, 1999: 183–261.

52. Hayakawa K, Hardy RR. Normal, autoimmune, and malignant CD5+ B cells: the Ly-1 B lineage? *Annu Rev Immunol* 1988; 6:197–218.

53. Hayakawa K, Hardy RR, Herzenberg LA. Progenitors for Ly-1 B cells are distinct from progenitors for other B cells. *J Exp Med* 1985; 161:1554–1568.

54. Hayakawa K, Hardy RR, Parks DR, Herzenberg LA. The 'Ly-1 B' cell subpopulation in normal immunodefective, and autoimmune mice. *J Exp Med* 1983; 157:202–218.

55. Antin JH, Emerson SG, Martin P, Gadol N, Ault KA. Leu-1+ (CD5+) B cells. A major lymphoid subpopulation in human fetal spleen: phenotypic and functional studies. *J Immunol* 1986; 136:505–510.

56. Casali P, Notkins AL. CD5+ B lymphocytes, polyreactive antibodies and the human B-cell repertoire. *Immunol Today* 1989; 10: 364–368.

57. Fischer M, Küppers R. Human IgA- and IgM-secreting intestinal plasma cells carry heavily mutated Vh region genes. *Eur J Immunol* 1998; 28:2971–2977.

58. Dunn-Walters DK, Boursier L, Spencer J. Hypermutation, diversity and dissemination of human intestinal lamina propria plasma cells. *Eur J Immunol* 1997; 27:2959–2964.

59. Boursier L, Dunn-Walters DK, Spencer J. Characteristics of IgVH genes used by human intestinal plasma cells from childhood. *Immunology* 1999; 97:558–564.

60. Macpherson AJ, Lamarre A, McCoy K, *et al.* IgA B cell and IgA antibody production in the absence of mu and delta heavy chain expression early in B cell ontogeny. *Nature Immunol* 2001; 2:625–631.

Modification of host cell function by normal flora – a molecular perspective

Andrew J Stagg

6

Introduction

Human beings harbour a complex and abundant ensemble of microbes. There are an estimated 2–4 million genes in these bacteria, compared with the 35,000 or so in our own genome. Bacteria have inhabited the Earth for at least 2.5 billion years,[1] but the ways in which coevolution of our ancestors with their indigenous microorganisms have shaped our physiology is poorly understood. Relationships between the human host and non-pathogenic bacteria are likely to include interactions that are symbiotic, where at least one partner benefits without harming the other, and commensal, where there is coexistence without detriment but without obvious benefit to either partner.[2] Most of our bacterial symbionts and commensals reside in our intestine[3] and so it is here where microorganisms are likely to have the most pronounced effects on our biology.

Much of what is regarded as normal gut structure and function is probably the end-point of interactions between the host and the microbes colonising the intestine (reviewed in Stagg *et al.*[4]). Studies in germ-free animals indicate that bacteria affect gut morphology,[5,6] motility,[7] epithelial differentiation[8] and immune system constituents.[9,10]

In vitro models using cultured intestinal cells can demonstrate a modulating effect of bacteria. For instance, non-virulent *Salmonella* strains are able to attenuate epithelial cell production of inflammatory cytokines by interfering with the NFκB signalling pathway.[11] However, these *in vitro* systems probably do not reflect the true complexity of events *in vivo*. Recently, a simplified mouse model system has been developed by J. Gordon and colleagues to allow the molecular analysis of the interactions between gut commensals and their host *in vivo*.[12] Some of the findings in this model are discussed below, and the reader is also referred to reference[12] for more detailed information.

Colonisation of germ-free mice with *Bacteroides thetaiotaomicron*

In the model, male germ-free mice were colonised with *Bacteroides thetaiotaomicron,* which is a prominent member of the murine and human ileal and colonic microflora. Normally this anaerobe colonises during the suckling/weaning transition, a time of rapid and pronounced functional maturation of the gut.[13] For experimental purposes, this organism also has the advantages that it can be cultured and can be genetically manipulated. Two approaches were used to analyse the

influence of colonisation on the transcription of host genes.[12] First, high-density Affymetrix Gene-Chips representing ~25,000 mouse genes were probed with cRNA prepared from total ileal RNA extracts from male germ-free and from aged-matched germ-free mice colonised 10 days previously with *B. thetaiotaomicron*. Second, to define the cellular origins of some host responses, laser-capture microdissection (LCM) of frozen ileal sections and real-time quantitative reverse transcriptase polymerase chain reactions ('Taqman' analyses) were used to compare gene expression in crypt and villus epithelium.

Changes in host gene expression following colonisation with *B. thetaiotaomicron*

In the Affymetrix analysis, pairwise comparisons of 'germ-free' and 'colonised' expression levels were performed.[12] All colonised mice had $\geq 10^7$ *B. thetaiotaomicron* cfu per millilitre of ileal contents. Changes of two-fold or greater were considered significant as long as the analysis software determined the mRNA to be present in either sample and that differences were observed in duplicate microarray hybridisations.

In this way, mRNAs represented by 118 probe sets changed two-fold or more following colonisation. Of these, 95 were increased and 23 decreased. Seventy-one genes were assigned to functional groups, whereas 34 transcripts were from uncharacterised genes.

Potential effects on nutrient uptake

Germ-free rodents require a 30% higher calorific intake than those with a microflora in order to maintain their body weight.[14] It is known that *Bacteroides* are able to hydrolyse dietary carbohydrates. The resulting monosaccharides provide a carbon source for the bacteria but can also be delivered to the host. The microarray analysis performed by Gordon *et al.* provides interesting clues about how *B. thetaiotaomicron* can enhance nutrient uptake by the host. Colonisation was associated with increased ileal expression of the mRNA for the Na+/glucose cotransporter (SGLT-1), which presumably facilitates host absorption. Concerted increases in several components of the host's lipid absorption machinery were also observed: colipase was increased up to 10-fold after colonisation, and LCM analysis indicated expression predominately in pannus cells at the crypt base. Pancreatic lipase-related protein 2 (PLRP-2) was also increased, which might be predicted to result in increased hydrolysis of triacylglycerides. Also upregulated were a fatty acid-binding protein (L-FABP) and apolipoprotein A-IV, which is involved in the packaging of complex lipids. The decreased expression of fasting-induced adipose factor

(PPARα), which is usually repressed by fat feeding,[15] provides further evidence for increased lipid uptake in colonised mice.

Potential effects on barrier function and metabolism of toxins

The most dramatic response to *B. thetaiotaomicron* was a 200-fold increase in expression of small proline-rich protein-2 (sprr2a). Members of the sprr family have been intensely studied in skin and contribute to the barrier function of squamous epithelium, both as a component of the cornified cell envelope and as a cross-bridging protein linked to desmosomal desmoplakin.[16] LCM/Taqman analysis indicated expression in the villus rather than the crypt, with a 280-fold increase in expression in the villus epithelium. Thus, it seems likely that sprr2a plays a role in fortifying the intestinal epithelial barrier in response to bacterial colonisation. Interestingly, although colonisation with *B. thetaiotaomicron* or the whole intestinal flora upregulated sprr2a, colonisation with *E. coli* or Bifidobacteria did not, indicating differences between bacteria species in their interaction with the host.

Dietary constituents and drugs are detoxified in the intestine by oxidation or conjugation. Colonisation with *B. thetaiotaomicrona* affected the expression of three host genes that are likely to participate in this detoxification process. Colonisation produced a twofold decrease in expression of glutathione S-transferase, which detoxifies electrophiles by conjugation to glutathione, and a fourfold decrease in multidrug resistance protein 1a (Mdr1a), which exports glutathione conjugated compounds from the epithelium.[17] Debrisoquine hydroxylase (CYP2D2), which is involved in oxidative drug metabolism in humans,[18] also declined threefold. Again, there were differences between bacterial species: colonisation with *E. coli* or Bifidobacteria resulted in an increase, rather than a decrease, in Mdr1a.

Effects on the immune system

Colonisation with *B. thetaiotaomicron* resulted in an influx of IgA-producing B cells, accompanied by increased expression of the polymeric immunoglobulin receptor (pIgR) that transports multimeric IgA across the epithelium. Decay-accelerating factor (DAF) was increased fivefold after colonisation, and may help prevent the activation of complement components in intestinal secretions that could result in damage to the mucosa. There was also augmented expression of the CRP-ductin, the product of which may act as a receptor for trefoil peptides.[19,20]

There was no change in members of the NFκB pathway of immune activation, possibly reflecting the need of the organism to avoid overt immune activation if it is to coexist successfully with the host.

Colonisation with whole flora results in more activation of immune system-associated genes than with *B. thetaiotaomicron*, perhaps suggesting that some bacterial species are able to actively downregulate or silence immune responses.

Other genes

Colonisation increased the expression of angiogenin-3, a poorly characterised secreted angigenesis factor, and angiogenin-related protein, which has no known angiogenic activity.[21,22] LCM/Taqman analysis revealed that the expression of angiogenin-3 was largely confined to the crypt epithelium, and here it is strategically placed to play a role in a number of host responses including nutrient absorption and, potentially, carcinogenesis. A potential effect of colonisation on motility is suggested by changes in expression of two components of the GABA-containing subpopulation of enteric neurons: L-glutamate decarboxylase (a glutamate transporter) and vesicle-associated protein 33 (a protein associated with granules produced in the ENS).

Discussion

The reductionist approach of colonisation with a single organism, developed by Gordon and colleagues using *B. thetaiotaomicron*, elegantly demonstrates the potential for modulation of expression of a wide range of host genes by a member of the intestinal flora. Whether all of the effects observed upon single-species colonisation of adult germ-free mice (in which intestinal development has proceeded somewhat abnormally in the absence of a flora) also occur during natural colonisation, from birth, with a complex flora, remains to be determined. However, it is already clear that introduction of a complex flora has many effects on host genes, and that these are likely to represent the net effect of the outcomes of multiple interactions between the host and different bacterial species. Comparison between different inbred mouse strains will determine whether, as seems likely, host genetic factors can be demonstrated to influence these interactions.

It is also becoming clear that spatial resolution within intestinal tissue is a critical part of such analyses. Analysis of tissues outside the intestinal mucosa will also inform about the 'long-range' effects of colonisation. Sites of interest could include the liver, vessel endothelia, and non-intestinal mucosal sites such as the lung.

Another important question is 'what bacterial products regulate the expression of host genes?' Currently, it is not even known whether viable *B. thetaiotaomicron* is required to produce the effects observed in germ-free mice. It is anticipated that sequencing of the 5.5 megabase genome of *B. thetaiotaomicron* will be complete by the end of 2001. This, together with systems for genetic

manipulation of the organism, should enable the identification of some of the bacterial molecules that interact with the host to alter gene expression. These tools will at last enable a much greater understanding of host–flora interactions at a molecular level.

References

1. Brocks JJ, Logan GA, Buick R, Summons RE. Archean molecular fossils and the early rise of eukaryotes. *Science* 1999; 285:1033–1036.

2. Hooper LV, Gordon JI. Commensal host-bacterial relationships in the gut. *Science* 2001; 292:1115–1118.

3. Savage DC. Microbial ecology of the gastrointestinal tract. *Annu Rev Microbiol* 1977; 31:107–133.

4. Falk PG, Hooper LV, Midtvedt T, Gordon JI. Creating and maintaining the gastrointestinal ecosystem: what we know and need to know from gnotobiology. *Microbiol Mol Biol Rev* 1998; 62:1157–1170.

5. Alam M, Midtvedt T, Uribe A. Differential cell kinetics in the ileum and colon of germfree rats. *Scand J Gastroenterol* 1994; 29:445–451.

6. Gustafsson BE, Midtvedt T, Strandberg K. Effects of microbial contamination on the cecum enlargement of germfree rats. *Scand J Gastroenterol* 1970; 5:309–314.

7. Husebye E, Hellstrom PM, Midtvedt T. Intestinal microflora stimulates myoelectric activity of rat small intestine by promoting cyclic initiation and aboral propagation of migrating myoelectric complex. *Dig Dis Sci* 1994; 39:946–956.

8. Bry L, Falk P, Huttner K, Ouellette A, Midtvedt T, Gordon JI. Paneth cell differentiation in the developing intestine of normal and transgenic mice. *Proc Natl Acad Sci USA* 1994; 91:10335–10339.

9. Guy-Grand D, Griscelli C, Vassalli P. The mouse gut T lymphocyte, a novel type of T cell. Nature, origin, and traffic in mice in normal and graft-versus-host conditions. *J Exp Med* 1978; 148:1661–1677.

10. Macpherson AJ, Gatto D, Sainsbury E, Harriman GR, Hengartner H, Zinkernagel RM. A primitive T cell-independent mechanism of intestinal mucosal IgA responses to commensal bacteria. *Science* 2000; 288:2222–2226.

11. Neish AS, Gewirtz AT, Zeng H, *et al.* Prokaryotic regulation of epithelial responses by inhibition of IkappaB- alpha ubiquitination. *Science* 2000; 289:1560–1563.

12. Hooper LV, Wong MH, Thelin A, Hansson L, Falk PG, Gordon JI. Molecular analysis of commensal host-microbial relationships in the intestine. *Science* 2001; 291:881–884.

13. Moore WEC, Holdeman LV. Human fecal flora: the normal flora of 20 Japanese-Hawaiians. *Appl Microbiol* 1974; 27:961–979.

14. Wostmann BS, Larkin C, Moriarty A, Bruckner-Kardoss E. Dietary intake, energy metabolism, and excretory losses of adult male germfree Wistar rats. *Lab Anim Sci* 1983; 33: 46–50.

15. Kersten S, Mandard S, Tan NS, *et al.* Characterization of the fasting-induced adipose factor FIAF, a novel peroxisome proliferator-activated receptor target gene. *J Biol Chem* 2000; 275:28488–28493.

16. Steinert PM, Marekov LN. Initiation of assembly of the cell envelope barrier structure of stratified squamous epithelia. *Mol Biol Cell* 1999; 10:4247–4261.

17. Johnstone RW, Ruefli AA, Smyth MJ. Multiple physiological functions for multidrug transporter P- glycoprotein? *Trends Biochem Sci* 2000; 25:1–6.

18. Ingelman-Sundberg M, Oscarson M, McLellan RA. Polymorphic human cytochrome P450 enzymes: an opportunity for individualised drug treatment. *Trends Pharmacol Sci* 1999; 20:342–349.

19. De Lisle RC, Petitt M, Isom KS, Ziemer D. Developmental expression of a mucinlike glycoprotein (MUCLIN) in pancreas and small intestine of CF mice. *Am J Physiol* 1998; 275:G219–G227.

20. Thim L, Mortz E. Isolation and characterization of putative trefoil peptide receptors. *Regul Pept* 2000; 90:61–68.

21. Fu X, Kamps MP. E2a-Pbx1 induces aberrant expression of tissue-specific and developmentally regulated genes when expressed in NIH 3T3 fibroblasts. *Mol Cell Biol* 1997; 17:1503–1512.

22. Fu X, Roberts WG, Nobile V, Shapiro R, Kamps MP. mAngiogenin-3, a target gene of oncoprotein E2a-Pbx1, encodes a new angiogenic member of the angiogenin family. *Growth Factors* 1999; 17:125–137.

Bacteria and the regulation of T-cell immune function in the gut

Thomas T MacDonald and Giovanni Monteleone

7

Introduction

The human intestinal immune system faces three quite distinct challenges. The first is the biomass of the complex resident microflora, which is clearly immunogenic, but against which it is not desirable to generate an excessive immune response because the consequence is chronic inflammation. The second is the large family of enteric bacterial pathogens, a response against which is needed in many cases to ensure host survival, but which has developed strategies to manipulate host immune responses in the gut wall. The third is that there is an imperative to remain functionally unresponsive to food protein antigens. In addition, all protective immune responses in the gut wall must take place in the face of a large amount of noise from the ongoing immune responses to the normal microflora. The mucosal immune system does not have the option of ignoring antigens, as T- and B-cell antigen receptors can only recognise non-self and cannot distinguish between a peptide from a member of the normal flora and that of a pathogen. It is often stated that the gut is an immunologically unresponsive site, but this is incorrect. In normal individuals the intestine is a site of intense immunological activity and the challenge is to maintain a disease-free state in the face of chronic antigen exposure. This is reflected in the huge amount of IgA produced in the gut (5 g/day) and the abundant T cells in the lamina propria and epithelium of healthy individuals.

The relationship between the normal flora and the mucosal immune system in normal individuals

No studies to date have shown that IgA is involved in protecting against the normal flora. Thus systemic infections with gut bacteria are not seen in IgA-deficient animals or humans. In contrast, animals or patients with defects in systemic non-specific immunity in neutrophils and macrophages suffer from systemic gut-derived infections, despite having normal mucosal T and B cells.[1,2]

The T-cell system of the gut is also in a constant state of activation in response to the normal flora. For example, germ-free animals have virtually no intraepithelial or lamina propria T cells.[3] Intraepithelial lymphocyte (IEL) numbers are clearly influenced by the flora, but in normal animals and in humans, they appear to be quite long-lived,[4] with a markedly skewed oligoclonal T-cell receptor repertoire[5] and there is little evidence that IEL are involved in gut disease. In contrast, the whole lamina propria T-cell population (mostly CD4+) appears to be renewed every 10–14 days in parabiotic rodents,[6] and studies tracking the fate of radiolabelled gut homing T blasts suggest that in fact the population may turn over every few days.[7] This suggests that there is not only massive death of T cells in the gut lamina propria, but that there must also be constant emigration of lamina propria homing T-cell blasts from the Peyer's patches. In the absence of T cells, there is again little evidence of excess penetration and persistence of normal flora in systemic tissues. Even mice without T or B cells survive with a normal flora as long as they are kept in a specific pathogen-free environment, but succumb rapidly when exposed to even low-grade pathogens.

We can therefore conclude from murine studies that although the normal bacterial flora elicits an enormous mucosal T- and B-cell response, this is of no functional significance for the gut bacteria themselves; in its absence, the bacteria of the normal flora do not invade the tissues. Teleologically it is probably the price that has to be paid in order to be able to respond to life-threatening gut pathogens. It has to be remembered that the immune system is inherently wasteful: there is massive cell division and death in the thymus and germinal centres for example.

The normal flora influences immune responses to bystander food antigens

It has long been recognised that germ-free animals show defects in cellular immunity. For example, one of the authors showed many years ago that germ-free mice showed defective cell-mediated immunity,[8] which is now explainable in terms of a deficiency in the Th1-inducing cytokine interleukin-12. However, in the gut of normal individuals the Peyer's patches (PPs) of the small bowel, and the colonic follicles and appendix are constantly exposed to an abundance of microbial products, transported across the follicle associated epithelium by M cells to antigen-presenting cells. Subepithelial dendritic cells (DCs) will almost certainly express toll-like receptors (TLRs), although this has not yet been studied in humans or animals. Peptidoglycans and lipoproteins from Gram-positive bacteria can activate DCs through TLR2. Lipopolysaccharide from Gram-negative organisms can activate through TLR4 and CpG DNA through TLR9.[9] Although the interest in TLRs has arisen through their role as pathogen recognition molecules, in the gut with an abundant indigenous microbial flora, there is no reason why peptidoglycans, lipopolysaccharide and lipoteichoic acids from this source should not also be capable of acting as ligands for TLRs. Engagement of TLRs by products of the normal flora would then activate nuclear factor (NF)-κB and the p38 mitogen-activated protein kinase via the adapter protein MyD88, and so increase IL-12 production.[9] Indeed we have shown in humans that IL-12-producing cells are located in the PP immediately below the dome epithelium.[10] Consistent with high local expression of IL-12, T cells in human PP show strongly biased Th1 responses to food antigens[10] and constitutive STAT4 activation.[11] This concept is illustrated in Figure 7.1.

The realisation that products of the normal flora might regulate the cytokine environment within PP and thus dictate the type of T-cell response generated to protein antigens has major implications. It is now virtually a dogma that mucosal T-cell responses are Th2/Th3 biased. However, most of these data have been generated in mice.[12,13] In contrast, in humans nearly all of the data suggest that mucosal T-cell responses are Th1 biased.[14] Differences between human and rodent mucosal immune responses may be related to the intestinal flora, which is markedly different between the two species. The human ileum has an abundant and diverse indigenous microflora,[15,16] and even in the upper bowel, where there are fewer PPs, *Helicobacter pylori* in the stomach of many individuals, oral microbes and microbes in foods must also be transported in the jejunal follicles. In contrast, mice often have a limited, specific pathogen-free flora, are often

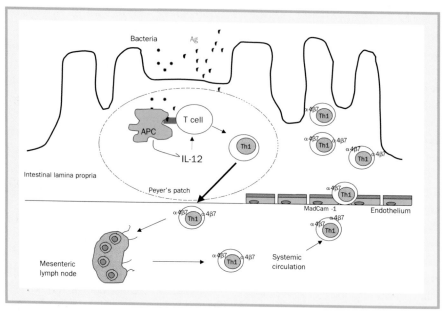

Figure 7.1
Gut bacteria activate antigen-presenting cells (APC) in PP to secrete IL-12. This then skews T-cell responses in the PP along the Th1 pathway, and these cells migrate to the lamina propria using α4β7 integrin/MAdCAM interactions to extravasate from the blood.

fed sterile food, and are usually used at a young age. For example the gold-standard mouse flora is the altered Schaedler Flora (ASF), which consists of only eight bacteria selected for low immunogenicity. Four are "fusiform-shaped" anaerobes and two are lactobacilli (*L. acidophilus* and *L. salivarius*); there is a spirochete-shaped anaerobe and a *Bacteroides distasonis.*[17] It is possible that mice with a limited flora are relatively deficient in

IL-12, so that their Th1 responses are compromised. Quantitative changes in the gut flora therefore may have profound effects on the cytokine environment in PPs, which in turn will have effects on the type of T-cell response generated to oral antigens. Of particular relevance is the explosion of atopic and allergic disease seen in the developed world in countries with a high standard of domestic hygiene. Newborn infants have a

Th2-biased immune system.[18] Early in life, it is thought that in most individuals, exposure to gut bacteria and pathogens switches this response to a Th1 type, perhaps through induction of IL-12. In the absence of childhood infections and a generally clean environment this switch does not occur, so that Th2 responses persist, with disease-causing consequences.

Normal intestinal bacteria can drive chronic gut inflammation

Four strands of evidence have now contributed to show that, in Crohn's disease, the antigens that drive the strongly polarised Th1 tissue-damaging response are derived from the normal bacterial flora. First, definitive proof of concept has come from studies of the multitude of models of inflammatory bowel disease seen in animals with dysregulated immune systems. In cases where it has been examined, the lesions are dependent on the presence of a normal flora, and in its absence there is no disease. Moreover, in some models, colonisation with normal flora rapidly results in T cell-mediated gut inflammation.[19] Second, strong circumstantial evidence comes from studies of patients with defects in phagocyte killing of bacteria, such as children with chronic granulomatous disease or glycogen storage disease type 1b. A subgroup of these children develop a disease similar to Crohn's disease.

Importantly, however, when the phagocyte defect is treated, the gut lesions resolve.[20,21] Third, it has been demonstrated that T cells from the lamina propria of Crohn's patients respond *in vitro* to the antigens of their own flora with a Th1 polarised response.[22] Finally, looser circumstantial evidence comes from patients in whom diversion of the faecal stream after surgery prevents the recurrence of Crohn's disease, and exposing the bowel to faecal contents results in inflammation.[23] The use of metronidazole to treat distal Crohn's disease,[24] and the fact that the disease occurs most often where gut bacteria are most abundant, also support a role for bacteria in driving inflammation. Taken together, this evidence is as close to Koch's postulates for proof of causation as is likely to be obtained. Attention is turning towards the ways in which gut bacteria can drive IL-12 production in the lamina propria, which can prevent the death of T cells sensitised to antigens of the normal flora (Figure 7.2).

In the context of probiotics it is extremely interesting that Gram-positive bacteria, including some lactobacilli, are extremely potent inducers of IL-12 in human monocytes.[25] It is thus possible that giving patients large amounts of lactobacilli might boost mucosal IL-12, which is probably not a good idea in Crohn's disease, although it may be useful in promoting Th2→Th1 skewing in the neonate and so prevent atopy. On the other hand, it would seem reasonable that

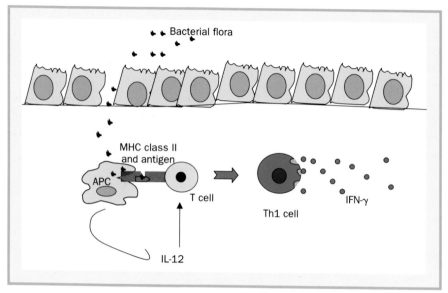

Figure 7.2
In Crohn's disease gut bacteria may cross a leaky epithelium and cause lamina propria antigen-presenting cells to secrete IL-12. This then drives Th1 cells to make interferon-γ and promote excess Th1 responses in the lamina propria.

reducing the bacterial flora in general by, for example, antibiotics, might downregulate IL-12 production, which may be of benefit in Crohn's disease.

Modifying specific intestinal bacteria to modulate local intestinal immunity

A great deal of excitement has been aroused by the recent observation that *Lactococcus lactis*, genetically engineered to make IL-10, was of therapeutic benefit in dextran sodium sulphate colitis and in the colitis seen in IL-10[-/-] mice.[26] Although these data are of interest, the experiment compared the IL-10-secreting organism with a control *L. lactis*, which had no effect. The crucial question is whether the IL-10-secreting *L. lactis* is actually more effective than *Lactobacillus reuteri* which is efficacious in mouse colitis.[27] This is an exciting development, but its use in humans will need to be judged on the success or failure of standard probiotic therapies in Crohn's and ulcerative colitis. Overall, however, this approach shows that it may be possible to genetically manipulate intestinal microbes to deliver immunomodulatory molecules into inflamed gut. In this regard, rather than targeting mammalian molecules, it may be more appropriate to focus on molecules made by intestinal pathogens which subvert gut immunity, as they have been selected by evolutionary pressure to produce function mucosal immune down-regulation. There are now many examples of these molecules:

- Sip B from virulent *Salmonella* is involved in the activation of caspase 2 in macrophages, which then induces apoptosis.[28]
- Non-virulent *Salmonella* prevent the ubiquitinisation of activated IκB.[29]
- YopJ of *Yersinia pseudotuberculosis* blocks cAMP response element-binding protein (CREB)-induced cellular and immune activation.[30]

Many of these molecules need to be injected into the mammalian cell by a type III secretion apparatus, which would not be appropriate for Gram-positive vectors but which could be engineered into commensal *E. coli*, for example. In the context of inflammatory bowel disease the focus is on strategies that downregulate mucosal immunity, but there are many contexts in which it may be desirable to boost mucosal

T-cell responses, such as vaccines. In this regard it is of interest that both *Yersinia* spp and enteropathic *E. coli* (EPEC) produce related molecules – invasin and intimin, respectively – which are potent activators of cell-mediated immunity.[31,32] This serves to reinforce the notion that the most potent modulators of immune response in the gut are those made by gut bacteria themselves.

References

1. Shiloh MU, MacMicking JD, Nicholson S, *et al.* Phenotype of mice and macrophages deficient in both phagocyte oxidase and inducible nitric oxide synthase. *Immunity* 1999; 10:29–38.

2. Johnston RB. Clinical aspects of chronic granulomatous disease. *Curr Opin Hematol* 2001; 8:17–22.

3. Guy-Grand D, Griscelli C, Vassalli P. The mouse gut T lymphocyte, a novel type of T cell. Nature origin, and traffic in mice in normal and graft-versus-host conditions. *J Exp Med* 1978; 148:1661–1677.

4. Penney LM, Kilshaw PJ, MacDonald TT. Regional variation in the proliferative rate and lifespan of alpha beta TCR⁺ and gamma delta TCR⁺ intraepithelial lymphocytes in the murine small intestine. *Immunology* 1995; 86:212–218.

5. Balk SP, Ebert EC, Blumenthal RL, *et al.* Oligoclonal expansion and Cd1 recognition by human intestinal intraepithelial lymphocytes. *Science* 1991; 253:1411–1415.

6. Poussier P, Edouard P, Lee C, Binnie M, Julius M. Thymus-independent development

and negative selection of T cells expressing T cell receptor alpha/beta in the intestinal epithelium: evidence for distinct circulation patterns of gut- and thymus-derived T lymphocytes. *J Exp Med* 1992; 176:187–199.

7. Parrott DMV, Lymphocyte recirculation outside the lymphoid system. In: Maria de Sousa, ed. *Lymphocyte Recirculation.* Chichester: John Wiley and Sons, 1981; 99–122.

8. MacDonald TT, Carter PB. Requirement for a bacterial flora before mice generate cells capable of mediating the delayed hypersensitivity reaction to sheep red blood cells. *J Immunol* 1979; 122:2426–2429.

9. Kaisho T, Akira S. Dendritic-cell function in Toll-like receptor and MyD88-knockout mice. *Trends Immunol* 2000; 22:78–83.

10. Nagata S, McKenzie C, Pender SL, *et al.* Human Peyer's patch T cells are sensitized to dietary antigen and display a T cell type 1 cytokine profile. *J Immunol* 2000; 165: 5315–5321.

11. Monteleone G, MacDonald TT. Interleukin 12 and Th1 immune responses in human Peyer's patches. *Trends Immunol* 2001; 22: 244–247.

12. Weiner HL, Oral tolerance: immune mechanisms and treatment of autoimmune diseases. *Immunol Today* 1997; 18:335–343.

13. Strobel S, Mowat AM. Immune responses to dietary antigens: oral tolerance. *Immunol Today* 1998; 19:173–181.

14. MacDonald TT. Effector and regulatory lymphoid cells and cytokines in mucosal sites. In: Neutra M, Kraehenbuhl J-P, eds. Defence of mucosal surfaces: pathogenesis, immunity and vaccines. *Curr Top Microbiol Immunol* 1999; 236:113–136.

15. Peach S, Lock MR, Katz D, *et al.* Mucosal-associated bacterial flora of the intestine in patients with Crohn's disease and in a control group. *Gut* 1978; 19:1043–1042.

16. Keighley MRB, Arabi Y, Dimock F, *et al.* Influence of inflammatory bowel disease on intestinal microflora. *Gut* 1978; 19: 1099–1104.

17. http://www.taconic.com/library/Culturing.

18. Martinez FD, Holt PG, Role of microbial burden in aetiology of allergy and asthma. *Lancet* 1999; 354(Suppl ii):12–15.

19. Sartor RB, Colitis in HLA-B27/beta 2 microglobulin transgenic rats. *Int Rev Immunol* 2000; 19:39–50.

20. Winkelstein JA, Marino MC, Johnston RB, *et al.* Chronic granulomatous disease. Report on a national registry of 368 patients. *Medicine* 2000; 79:155–169.

21. Roe TF, Coates TD, Thomas DW, *et al.* Treatment of chronic inflammatory bowel disease in glycogen storage disease type 1b with colony stimulating factors. *N Engl J Med* 1992; 326:1666–1669.

22. Duchmann R, Kaiser I, Herman E, *et al.* Tolerance exists towards resident intestinal flora but is broken in active inflammatory bowel disease. *Clin Exp Immunol* 1995; 102: 448–455.

23. D'Haens GR, Geboes K, Peeters M, *et al.* Early lesions of recurrent Crohn's disease caused by infusion of intestinal contents in excluded ileum. *Gastroenterology* 1998; 114: 262–267.

24. Rutgeerts P, Hiele M, Geboes K, *et al.* Controlled trial of metronidazole treatment for prevention of Crohn's recurrence after ileal resection. *Gastroenterology* 1995; 108: 1617–1621.

25. Miettinen M, Matikainen S, Vuopio-Varkila J, *et al.* Lactobacilli and streptococci induce IL-12, IL-18 and gamma-interferon production in human peripheral blood mononuclear cells. *Infect Immun* 1998; 66:6058–6062.

26. Steidler L, Hans W, Schotte L, *et al.* Treatment of murine colitis by *Lactococcus lactis* secreting IL-10. *Science* 2000; 289: 1352–1355.

27. Madsen KL, Doyle JS, Jewell LD, *et al. Lactobacillus* species prevents colitis in Il-10 gene-deficient mice. *Gastroenterology* 1999; 116:1107–1114.

28. Jesenberger V, Procyk KJ, Yuan J, *et al.* Salmonella-induced caspase 2 activation in macrophages: a novel mechanism in pathogen-mediated apoptosis. *J Exp Med* 2000; 192:1035–1046.

29. Neish AS, Gewirtz AT, Zeng H, *et al.* Prokaryotic regulation of epithelial responses by inhibition of IkappaB-alpha ubiquitination. *Science* 2000; 289:1560–1563.

30. Meijer LK, Schesser K, Wolf-Watz H, *et al.* The bacterial protein YopJ abrogates multiple signal transduction pathways that converge on the transcription factor CREB. *Cell Microbiol* 2000; 2:231–238.

31. Ennis E, Isberg RR, Shimizu Y. Very late antigen 4-dependent adhesion and costimulation of resting human T cells by the bacterial β1 integrin ligand invasin. *J Exp Med* 1993; 177:207–212.

32. Higgins LM, Frankel G, Connerton I, Goncalvez NS, Dougan G, MacDonald TT. Role of bacterial intimin in colonic hyperplasia and inflammation. *Science* 1999; 285:588–591.

Summary and observations

Thomas T Macdonald

Chapters 5–7 provide new insights into the relationship between the flora and host. The common theme is that there is a major functional relationship between intestinal microbes, the gut epithelium and the gut immune system, and that we know virtually nothing about the mechanisms involved. From first principles this is obvious. The gut has an epithelial surface area of 400 m^2; it also contains more lymphoid tissue (intraepithelial lymphocytes, lamina propria lymphocytes, Peyer's patches, solitary follicles and colonic follicles) than the rest of the body combined; and the ileum and colon are host to over 400 species of bacteria comprising 10^{14} organisms, many of which are uncharacterized and unculturable. In the 1960s, with the development of gnotobiotic technology, it became clear that the major stimulus for the development of the mucosal immune system, serum antibodies and digestive enzymes was the normal flora.

Gnotobiotic laboratories were relatively widespread in the 1960s and 1970s, but their high running cost and the absence of a clear vision of how gnotobiotic animals could help medical research led to the closure of the majority of these facilities. However, in the 1990s, the normal flora was again put back in the mainstream when its major role in the development of chronic inflammatory bowel disease was recognized thanks to new developments in molecular techniques and molecular immunology, and some understanding was gained of the myriad ways that mammals have evolved to recognize bacterial products.

The work performed by Jeffrey Gordon's group, and discussed in Chapter 6, has explored the modification of host cell function by the normal flora. The reductionist approach of colonization with a single organism, *Bacteroides thetaiotaomicron*, elegantly demonstrates the potential for modulation of expression of a wide range of host genes by a member of the intestinal flora. Whether all of the effects observed upon single-species colonization of adult germ-free mice (in which intestinal development has proceeded somewhat abnormally in the absence of a flora) also occur during natural colonization, from birth, with a complex flora, remains to be determined. However, it is already clear that introduction of a complex flora has many effects on host gene expression, and that these are likely to represent the net effect of the outcomes of multiple interactions between the host and different bacterial species. Comparison between different inbred mouse strains will determine whether, as seems likely, host genetic factors can be demonstrated to influence these interactions.

It is also becoming clear from Gordon's work that spatial resolution within intestinal tissue is a critical part of such analyses. Responses in the colon do not necessarily reflect those in the ileum. These findings suggest that a 'genome anatomy' analysis of the different regions of the intestine is likely to prove very interesting. Analysis of tissues outside the intestinal mucosa will also inform about 'long-range' effects of colonization. Sites of interest could include the liver, vessel endothelia and non-intestinal mucosal sites, such as the lung.

Another important question is, 'What bacterial products regulate expression of host genes?' Currently, it is not even known whether viable *B. thetaiotaomicron* is required to produce the effects observed in germ-free mice. It is anticipated that sequencing of the 5.5 megabase genome of *B. thetaiotaomicron* will be complete by the end of 2001. This, together with systems for genetic manipulation of the organism, should enable the identification of some of the bacterial molecules that interact with the host to alter gene expression. These tools will at last lead to a much greater understanding of host–flora interactions at a molecular level.

Despite the immense density of bacteria in the lower intestine of mammals, it is relatively unusual for intestinal or systemic problems to occur, at least in healthy individuals or when immunocompetent experimental animals are housed in a specific pathogen-free facility. This is hardly surprising, since vertebrates have co-evolved with their commensal intestinal bacterial flora, and so are adept at confining most of the flora to the intestinal lumen and highly efficient at clearing bacteria that penetrate the mucosal barrier.

In mice the normal flora elicits a secretory IgA response. The work described in Chapter 5 shows that this antibody response has a significant T-cell-independent component and also occurs in the absence of Peyer's patches. Although generated from peritoneal B1 cells, this response is different from the so-called natural antibodies made by B1 cells in that it is antigen-specific and can be elicited by luminal administration of bacterial proteins. Where B1 cells committed to make this IgA response encounter gut bacterial antigens is not known. Likewise, it is unclear whether this IgA response against the bacterial flora plays a role in preventing the bacteria from crossing the mucosal barrier.

Assessing animal and human models go hand in hand, but it needs to be remembered that there are major species differences. Indeed, even the existence of the B1 population of cells, studied by Macpherson in the mouse, is contentious in humans. Furthermore, Chapter 7 describes a study on human Peyer's patches that indicates a significant difference between rodents and humans. Chapter 7 argues that Peyer's patches are clearly a Th1-dominated environment in humans, unlike the situation in rodents. This Th1 dominance is most probably due to molecules from the normal flora crossing the FAE and inducing IL-12 in subepithelial dendritic cells. The presence of IL-12 then sets the conditions in which responses to food proteins become skewed along the Th1 pathway because IL-12 activates STAT-4. The Peyer's patches are therefore a sump of potentially tissue-damaging Th1 cells responding to myriads of antigens of the flora and food proteins. In healthy individuals these cells migrate to the lamina propria and probably die, but in food sensitive enteropathy and Crohn's disease they re-encounter antigen in the lamina propria and drive inflammation. There has been much speculation that probiotic bacteria and prebiotics expressing immunosuppressive cytokines might offer a new therapeutic tool for IBD and food-sensitive enteropathies, but overcoming the biological activity of the normal flora might be more difficult than anticipated.

What could account for the differences between humans and laboratory rodents? Chapter 7 argues that the answer may lie in differences in intestinal flora. Humans are outbred: many have a pathogen/commensal (*Helicobacter pylori*) in their stomach and they have diverse flora. In contrast, mice from reputable vendors have a defined flora of only a few organisms chosen by Schaedler in the 1960s because of their low immunogenicity. Thus it is not surprising that there are major differences between immune responses in the intestines of mice and humans. There are also differences in signalling pathways. In humans, interferon-alpha signalling through the JAK/STAT pathway is a very potent activator of Th1 responses. However, in mice, this is not the case because of a minisatellite insertion in the gene that codes for STAT2 so that it is unable to recruit STAT4 into the interferon-alpha signalling complex. Despite these differences between mice and humans, paradigms of host–bacterial interactions in the gut need to be established in animal models to produce hypotheses that are testable in humans.

There is a clear resonance between the elegant work demonstrating that the normal flora controls gene expression in the gut epithelium, and the work suggesting that in humans the over-expression of IL-12 in Peyer's patches (traditionally thought to be the inductive site of mucosal immune responses) is also due to the bioactivity of the flora. Thus the flora conditions gene expression in the two most important compartments of the gut involved in absorption and host defence, and it is reasonable to ask if this is an accident or a coevolutionary tactic. Chapter 5 effectively characterizes the existence of a primitive secretory IgA response in mice. The paradox of this response, however, is that even though it is elicited by the flora, it does not appear to have any obvious effect. This, however, depends on our ability to ask questions about the micro-ecology of the flora, and it may be that this IgA response is crucially important, but in unexpected ways (either for the host or the bacteria).

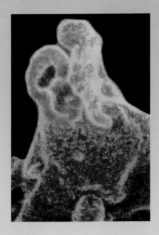

PART 3
Food, prebiotics and bacteria

Coeliac disease: a model to study oral tolerance

Olle Hernell, Göte Forsberg, Sten Hammarström, Anneli Ivarsson and Marie-Louise Hammarström

8

Introduction

Food-allergic diseases are features of childhood and may represent a breakdown or failure of oral tolerance induction or maintenance. While most food-allergic diseases are self-limiting, coeliac disease is characterized by a permanent intolerance to gluten. In genetically predisposed individuals, wheat gluten and related proteins in barley and rye may cause an inflammatory small bowel enteropathy that resolves with a gluten-free diet. The enzyme tissue transglutaminase was recently suggested to be the main autoantigen in coeliac disease. Coeliac disease has many similarities to autoimmune diseases, but differs in that the disease can be shut off by withdrawal of a known antigen from the diet. Hence, coeliac disease could be a useful model for studies of oral tolerance as well as autoimmunity.

In this chapter we review our experience from the Swedish epidemic of coeliac disease in children under 2 years of age, and provide evidence that oral tolerance to gluten is likely to be affected not only by early feeding practices but also by other environmental factors, supporting the view that the disease has a multifactorial aetiology. Using RNA from isolated intraepithelial and lamina propria T lymphocytes from freshly collected small intestinal biopsies and quantitative real-time reverse transcriptase polymerase chain reaction (RT-PCR), we studied the cytokine expression profiles in active and treated coeliac disease, respectively. We suggest that the small intestinal lesion is caused by an uncontrolled production of interferon-γ (IFN-γ) and a failure to produce a sufficient amount of transforming growth factor β1 (TGF-β1) to counteract the harmful effect of IFN-γ on the epithelium. We speculate that TGF-β1 provided by human milk could partly explain our observation that introducing gluten while the child is still breastfed reduces the risk of developing intolerance.

From the weaning period and onwards, the intestinal mucosa is exposed to an ever-increasing number of antigens, e.g. food components, microorganisms and various chemical substances. Only a minority of the foreign antigens that may reach the systemic circulation from the intestinal lumen is potentially harmful to humans and needs to be defended against. The vast majority of intestinal antigens do not require a protective immune response and may even be beneficial for the individual, e.g. dietary antigens. It follows that the intestinal mucosal immune system must have the capacity to discriminate between when an appropriate protective immune response to harmful foreign antigens is required and when a muted or non-response

to foreign antigens is preferable. One important component of the latter is oral tolerance, which may be defined as a systemic hyporesponsiveness or non-responsiveness of mature T and B cells to antigen challenge after prior oral exposure to that antigen, i.e. a decreased systemic immune response to antigens encountered previously by the mucosal immune system in the gut.[1,2]

Coeliac disease is defined as a permanent intolerance to gliadin in wheat gluten, and related prolamines in barley and rye, which causes an enteropathy in genetically susceptible individuals. In the coeliac patient, ingestion of such prolamines causes a lesion in the small intestinal mucosa characterized by an increased number of intraepithelial (IEL) and lamina propria (LPL) lymphocytes, crypt hyperplasia and villous atrophy.[3,4] When gluten (wheat, barley and rye) is eliminated from the diet the morphology of the mucosa is restored and the symptoms disappear.[3] Hence, gluten withdrawal is the current treatment for coeliac disease. Infants and young children generally develop a classic intestinal malabsorption syndrome within months after gluten is introduced into the diet, while less obvious symptoms are the rule rather than the exception in older children and adults.[5] The disease may present with extraintestinal symptoms, even in the absence of intestinal symptoms, or with symptoms due to associated disease, generally autoimmune in type, which points to coeliac disease being a type of autoimmune disease.[6] A recent population-based study of Swedish adults revealed a prevalence of 5.3 per 1000, of which 80% were undiagnosed prior to the study.[7]

More than 90% of patients with coeliac disease express the HLA class II DQ2 heterodimer, and most others the DQ8 molecule.[4] Recently, an association was also found with DR53.[8] However, other as yet unidentified genes are supposed to contribute at least as much to the genetic influence in coeliac disease. Several distinct T cell epitopes that bind to DQ2 and also DQ8 have been demonstrated within gluten.[4] Recently, Anderson *et al*.[9] suggested that the primary toxic epitope consists of 17 amino acid residues, of which glutamine 65 is deamidated to glutamic acid by the enzyme tissue transglutaminase (tTG), increasing the affinity for the DQ2 groove. tTG has also been defined as the major autoantigen in coeliac disease, and raised serum levels of particularly IgA antibodies to tTG, as well as to gliadin, the major prolamine in wheat gluten, and endomysium are used as markers of the disease,[6] although they may not be a prerequisite for the disease to develop. Thus, there are several good reasons why we believe that coeliac disease may help our understanding, not only of how oral tolerance is accomplished in humans, but also of the pathogenesis of autoimmune diseases. At least part of the genetics is known, the structures of

toxic epitopes that trigger the disease are known, the autoantibody is known, and the disease can be turned on and shut off by manipulating the diet.

A multi-factorial disease

It is a matter of debate to what extent environmental factors besides gluten influence the disease process.[10] We recently had a unique opportunity to study the impact of environmental exposure on the disease occurrence. From the mid-1980s Sweden experienced an epidemic of coeliac disease in the childhood population. After an initial threefold increase in incidence (to a highest level of 4.4 per 1000 born at 2 years of age, i.e. 1/227), there was a plateau, after which the incidence again rapidly decreased during the mid-1990s to the level preceding the epidemic.[11] The epidemic was restricted to children under 2 years of age, suggesting that early exposure, such as infant feeding patterns, might be an essential part of the explanation. Moreover, we believe that this type of epidemic curve is quite unique for a lifelong immunological disease with many similarities to autoimmune diseases.

To study the epidemic, we started a prospective incidence register based on 40% of the Swedish childhood population. All patients had their diagnosis verified by a small intestinal biopsy showing the typical enteropathy.[3] Based on this register, we carried out an incident case–referent study which focused on possible environmental risk factors. Dietary patterns in infancy differed significantly between cases diagnosed before 2 years of age and their referents.[12] The median duration of breast-feeding was 7 months for referents compared to 5 months for cases. A significantly larger proportion of referents were still being breastfed when gluten-containing foods were introduced into the diet. The majority of children were introduced to flour at 5–6 months of age, although this was more common for cases than for referents. Cases received larger initial amounts of flour, assessed as the amount consumed daily 2 weeks after the first portion. Large in this context refers to the upper third of the range consumed by the referents. There were no significant differences with respect to early feeding practices in older children. Based on these descriptive data, we developed models for a tentative influence of dietary patterns on the risk for coeliac disease, and evaluated these by conditional logistic regression in bivariate and multivariate analyses. If the infant was breastfed at the time of gluten introduction, this reduced the risk for coeliac disease. If the infant continued to be breastfed beyond the introduction, this reduced the risk further. The introduction of gluten-containing foods at 5–6 months of age was associated with an increased risk compared with earlier or later introduction. Introduction with large rather than small or

medium amounts of gluten also increased the risk. Because of possible confounding owing to the fact that the components of dietary patterns are associated with one another, multivariate analyses were performed. This confirmed a protective effect of introducing gluten-containing foods when the infant is still breastfed, as illustrated by an odds ratio of 0.6. This effect is even more pronounced if breastfeeding is continued after the introduction of gluten. Furthermore, a large rather than a small or a medium consumption 2 weeks after the first portion increases the risk for disease, as illustrated by an odds ratio of 1.5. When controlling for the amount of gluten and breastfeeding, the age at introduction no longer remained an independent risk factor. These effects of early feeding pattern were only seen in the youngest age group, i.e. children up to 2 years of age.[12]

Other risk factors that we have identified so far include gender. Confirming previous studies, we found that coeliac disease is twice as common in girls as in boys. This gender difference remained throughout the epidemic. Another risk factor is the season of birth. To be born in the summer rather than the winter increases the risk by 40% in the youngest age group. Interestingly, infections seem to have opposite effect on coeliac disease compared with atopic disease. Two or more infections, excluding gastroenteritis, during the first 6 months of life increase the risk; the risk is further increased if infants having had two or more infections are also exposed to large amounts of gluten during its introduction.[13]

Mucosal immune responses to gluten exposure

It now seems clear that T lymphocytes play a key role in the pathogenesis of coeliac disease. The numbers of intraepithelial lymphocytes (IEL), both αβ and γδ T cells, are increased in the small intestinal mucosa of coeliac disease patients.[14–16] The number of both intraepithelial αβ T cells and activated CD4+ αβ T cells in lamina propria increases in active disease.[14,17] Gliadin-specific CD4+ αβ T-cell clones have been isolated from the small intestinal mucosa of patients with coeliac disease.[18] Interestingly, the disease was in fact transmitted from a female patient to her HLA-identical brother by transplantation of bone marrow containing T cells.[19] Gliadin-induced local T cell-dependent immune reactions in coeliac disease are further indicated by induction of anti-endomysium antibody secretion[20] and increased interferon-γ (IFN-γ) mRNA expression[21] after *ex vivo* gliadin challenge of small intestinal biopsies of patients with coeliac disease.

In order to understand the adaptive local immune reactions in coeliac disease, we set out to analyse the cytokine response of small intestinal T cells of coeliac patients to *in vivo* exposure to gluten. Small intestinal biopsies were taken as routine diagnostic procedure according to the ESPGHAN criteria,[22] and part of the material was used for the present study. Two groups of patients with active coeliac disease were investigated: newly diagnosed children who responded promptly to withdrawal of gluten from the diet, and children who reacted adversely on challenge with a normal gluten-containing diet after a symptom-free period on a gluten-free diet. Both groups had abnormal mucosa compatible with active coeliac disease. These were compared to coeliac disease patients who had been treated with gluten-free diet for at least 7 months and were without symptoms, and a group of infants with no known food intolerance. The latter two groups had normal mucosa morphology. Intraepithelial and lamina propria T lymphocytes were isolated separately, and cytokine mRNA levels in freshly isolated T cells (CD3+) were determined using quantitative RT-PCR. Interleukin-2 (IL-2), a key cytokine for T-cell responses, the Th1 cytokines interferon-γ (IFN-γ) and tumour necrosis factor-α (TNF-α), the Th2 cytokine IL-4, and the downregulatory cytokines IL-10 and transforming growth factor-β1 (TGF-β1) were analysed. The cytokine profile of intestinal T cells in the control group showed a great resemblance to that of IEL in normal small intestinal mucosa of adults with expression of IL-2, TNF-α, TGF-β1 and no detectable expression of IL-4. However, IFN-γ expression was low in children compared to adults. Active coeliac disease was characterized by highly significant increases in both IFN-γ and IL-10, and the proportional expression of IFN-γ relative to TGF-β1 was significantly increased. There was also a marked shift of IFN-γ and IL-10 mRNA expression from lamina propria T cells to intraepithelial T cells. Interestingly, intraepithelial T cells in symptom-free coeliac disease patients on a gluten-free diet still had elevated IFN-γ levels compared to controls. Notably, there were no increases in IL-2, TNF-α or TGF-β1 levels in active coeliac disease, and IL-4 was not induced. Experiments with subfractionated intraepithelial T cells of patients with active disease suggest that IFN-γ and IL-10 are produced by different T-cell subtypes, and that CD8⁺ αβ T cells constitute the main source of IFN-γ.

Taken together, these results suggest that children with coeliac disease respond to gluten intake by an overreaction in small intestinal intraepithelial T lymphocytes, which exhibit uncontrolled production of IFN-γ and IL-10. Both recruitment of CD8⁺ αβ IEL and a leaky epithelium may be the consequences of this, leading to a vicious circle with amplified immune activity and destruction of the intestinal mucosa. We hypothesize that the intestinal epithelial cells respond to gluten in the same way as they do to insults by pathogenic microorganisms, including the secretion of chemokines recruiting CD8⁺ αβ T cells that secrete IFN-γ as part of their protective effector mechanism. IFN-γ/TGF-β1 imbalance may cause escalation of inflammation by a decreased ability to turn off

T-cell activity, as well as failure to 'seal' the epithelium. TGF-β1 provided by human milk could, at least partly, explain the protective effect of introducing gluten while the mother is still breastfeeding.

References

1. Strobel S, Mowat A McI. Immune responses to dietary antigens: oral tolerance. *Immunol Today* 1998;19:173–181.

2. Spiekermann GM, Walker WA. Oral tolerance and its role in clinical disease. *J Pediatr Gastroenterol Nutr* 2001; 32:237–255.

3. Marsh MN. Gluten, major histocompatibility complex, and the small intestine. A molecular and immunobiologic approach to the spectrum of gluten sensitivity. *Gastroenterology* 1992; 102:330–354.

4. Sollid LM. Molecular basis of celiac disease. *Annu Rev Immunol* 2000; 18:53–81.

5. Ferguson A. Coeliac disease research and clinical practice: maintaining momentum into the twenty-first century. *Baillières Clin Gastroenterol* 1995; 9:395–412.

6. Schuppan D. Current concepts of coeliac disease pathogenesis. *Gastroenterology* 2000; 119:234–242.

7. Ivarsson A, Persson LÅ, Peltonen M, Suhr O, Hernell O. High prevalence of undiagnosed coeliac disease in adults: a Swedish population-based study. *J Intern Med* 1999; 245:63–68.

8. Clot F, Gianfrani C, Babron MC, *et al.* HLA-DR53 molecules are associated with susceptibility to coeliac disease and selectively bind gliadin-derived peptides. *Immunogenetics* 2000; 51:249–251.

9. Anderson RP, Degano P, Godkin AJ, Jewell DP, Hill AVS. In vivo challenge in coeliac

disease identifies a single transglutaminase-modified peptide as the dominant A-gliadin T-cell epitope. *Nature Med* 2000; 6:337–342.

10. Ivarsson A, Persson LÅ, Hernell O. Does breast-feeding affect the risk for coeliac disease? *Adv Exp Med Biol* 2000; 478: 139–149.

11. Ivarsson A, Persson LÅ, Nyström L, *et al.* Epidemic of coeliac disease in Swedish children. *Acta Paediatr* 2000; 89:165–171.

12. Ivarsson A, Hernell O, Stenlund H, Persson LÅ. Breast-feeding protects against coeliac disease. *Am J Clin Nutr* 2001 (in press).

13. Ivarsson A. On the multifactorial etiology of coeliac disease. An epidemiological approach to the Swedish epidemic. Doctoral Thesis 2001. Umeå University Medical Dissertations. New series 739.

14. Kutlu T, Brousse N, Rambaud C, Le Deist F, Schmitz J, Cerf-Bensussan N. Numbers of T cell receptor (TCR) αβ+ but not of TCR γδ+ intraepithelial lymphocytes correlate with the grade of villous atrophy in coeliac patients on a long term normal diet. *Gut* 1993; 34:208–214.

15. Savilahti E, Arato A, Verkasalo M. Intestinal γ/δ receptor-bearing T lymphocytes in celiac disease and inflammatory bowel diseases in children. Constant increase in coeliac disease. *Pediatric Res* 1990; 28:579–581.

16. Iltanen S, Holm K, Ashorn M, Ruuska T, Laippala P, Mäki M. Changing jejunal γδ T cell receptor (TCR)-bearing intraepithelial lymphocyte density in coeliac disease. *Clin Exp Immunol* 1999; 117:51–55.

17. Halstensen TS, Brandtzaeg P. Activated T lymphocytes in the coeliac lesion: non-proliferative activation (CD25) of CD4⁺ α/β cells in the lamina propria but proliferation (Ki-67) of α/β and γ/δ cells in the epithelium. *Eur J Immunol* 1993; 23:505–510.

18. Lundin KEA, *et al.* Gliadin-specific, HLA-DQ (α1*0501,β1*0201) restricted T cells isolated from the small intestinal mucosa of coeliac disease patients. *J Exp Med* 1993; 178:187–196.

19. Bargetzi MJ, Schonenberger A, Tichelli A, *et al.* Coeliac disease transmitted by allogeneic non-T cell-depleted bone marrow transplantation. *Bone Marrow Transplant* 1997; 20:607–609.

20. Picarelli A, Maiuri L, Frate A, Greco M, Auriccio S, Londei M. Production of antiendomysial antibodies after in-vitro challenge of small intestine biopsy samples from patients with coeliac disease. *Lancet* 1996; 348:1065–1067.

21. Nilsen E, Jahnsen FL, Lundin KEA, *et al.* Gluten induces an intestinal cytokine response strongly dominated by interferon-γ in patients with coeliac disease. *Gastroenterology* 1998; 115:551–563.

22. Meeuwisse GW. Diagnostic criteria in coeliac disease. European Society for Pediatric Gastroenterology, Interlaken, 1969. *Acta Paediatr Scand* 1970; 59:461–463.

Effects of prebiotics on human gut health

Glenn R Gibson

9

Introduction

Recent years have seen a major change in how the activity of the human gastrointestinal tract is perceived. This has been driven by increased knowledge of the gut microflora, composition and activities. In particular, the colon is the most heavily populated region of the gastrointestinal tract and, because of this resident microbiota, is the most metabolically active organ in the body. Many studies have focused on the pathological aspects of human gut microbiology, but the situation now is that more positive aspects are being realised and exploited.

The concept of modulating activities directed towards improving gut microbial function has a long history, but has never enjoyed the topicality that is now evident. Nutritionists and clinicians have recognised this biological potential, as diet can have a major effect on the gut microflora activity. The latest developments in functional food science have exploited the route of manipulating this microbiota for improved health.

The human gastrointestinal tract, principally the colon, is a site of intense microbial activity. From culture-based data it is thought that at least 500 different microbial species exist, although on a quantitative basis around 10–20 genera probably predominate. Examples include *Bacteroides, Lactobacillus, Clostridium, Fusobacterium, Bifidobacterium, Eubacterium, Peptococcus, Peptostreptococcus, Escherichia* and *Veillonella*.[1]

Although some indigenous bacteria can be pathogenic (e.g. proteolytic clostridia and *Bacteroides*) in nature, it is also the case that some species may offer health-promoting attributes. For example, bifidobacteria and lactobacilli are thought to exert powerful antipathogenic capabilities and are mainly responsible for 'colonisation resistance' in the gut. Moreover, the same genera have been attributed with other beneficial aspects, such as stimulation of the immune response (which has positive implications for atopy in children and irritable bowel syndrome in adults), protection from bowel tumours, and metabolism of cholesterol and other lipids in the gut.[1] Although many of the health-promoting aspects have yet to be definitively proven in humans, it would appear that there is great value in eliciting a change away from a gut flora dominated by potentially harmful bacteria towards a more benign, or beneficial, composition.

Probiotics

The most frequently used dietary method of influencing the composition of gut flora is that of probiotics, whereby live microbial additions are made to appropriate food vehicles, usually fermented milks.[2] The first recorded intake of deliberate bacterial consumption was over 2000 years ago. However, the situation was put on a scientific footing by the writings of Metchnikoff at the Pasteur Institute.[2] He hypothesised that longevity in Bulgarian peasants was associated with their elevated intake of 'soured milks', i.e. dairy-based drinks containing live bacteria. This was the basis of what is now recognised as the probiotic concept, whereby an array of dietary ingredients deliberately supplemented with microorganisms exists. A recent formal definition of probiotics was agreed by a working party of European scientists and given as 'a live microbial feed supplement that is beneficial to health'.[3]

Over the years many species of microorganisms have been used. These consist not only of lactic acid bacteria (lactobacilli, streptococci, enterococci, lactococci, bifidobacteria), but also *Bacillus* spp. and fungi such as *Saccharomyces* spp. and *Aspergillus* spp. The commonest probiotics belong to the genera *Lactobacillus* (e.g. *L. casei, L. acidophilus, L. rhamnosus, L. johnsonii, L. reuteri*) and *Bifidobacterium* (e.g. *B. bifidum, B. longum, B. breve*).

Probiotic trials should use the best methodologies available. One difficulty lies in the recovery of fed strains in faeces. Moreover, it would appear that a significant proportion of the human gut microbiota is 'non-culturable'. As such, there has been a recent move away from cultural procedures coupled with phenotypic (morphological, biochemical) assessments of culture identity, towards more sophisticated molecular procedures.[4] These include nucleic acid fingerprinting studies for reliable identification, as well as the development of genetic probing systems such that predominant components of the gut flora can be quantified in a culture-independent manner.

Prebiotics

An alternative, or additional, approach is the prebiotic concept. A prebiotic is a non-digestible food ingredient that beneficially affects the host by selectively stimulating the growth and/or activity of one or a limited number of bacteria in the colon that can improve health.[5] Thus, the prebiotic approach advocates the administration of non-viable entities. Dietary carbohydrates, such as fibre, are candidate prebiotics, but most promise has been realised with oligosaccharides. In particular, the ingestion of fructo-oligosaccharides has been shown to stimulate bifidobacteria in the lower gut. As prebiotics exploit non-viable food ingredients, their applicability in diets is wide ranging. A further approach is synbiotics, where probiotics and prebiotics are combined.[5] Here, survivability of the live microbial addition in the gastrointestinal tract would be enhanced by coupling it with a selective growth substrate.

The prebiotic activity of fructose-containing oligosaccharides has been confirmed in both laboratory and human trials.[6–10] This is because these carbohydrates have a specific colonic fermentation directed towards bifidobacteria – which are purported to have a number of health-promoting properties.[1,5] Bifidobacteria are able to breakdown and utilise fructo-oligosaccharides, owing to their possession of a β-fructofuranosidase enzyme, providing a competitive advantage in a mixed culture environment such as the human gut.[11]

Galacto-oligosaccharides (GOS) are another class of prebiotics that are manufactured and marketed in Europe as well as in Japan. These consist of a lactose core with one or more galactosyl residues linked via $\beta 1 \rightarrow 3$, $\beta 1 \rightarrow 4$ and $\beta 1 \rightarrow 6$ bonds.[12] They have found application in infant formula foods, as they are naturally present (albeit in very low quantities) in human milk.

A different class of galacto-oligosaccharides, used as prebiotics in Japan, are those isolated from soybean whey. These soybean oligosaccharides (SOS) are composed of galactosyl residues linked $\alpha 1 \rightarrow 6$ to a sucrose core.[12]

Gluco-oligosaccharides can also act as prebiotics. Isomalto-oligosaccharides (IMO) are comprised of glucosyl residues linked by

$\alpha1\rightarrow6$ bonds.[12] These oligosaccharides are only partially prebiotic, as they are metabolised by humans. They are, however, very slowly metabolised, and most isomalto-oligosaccharides in the diet would pass through to the colon.

Xylo-oligosaccharides (XOS) are also used as prebiotics in Japan. These consist of xylosyl residues linked by $\beta1\rightarrow4$ bonds[12] and are much more acid stable than other prebiotics. For this reason, they have found application in soft drinks that tend to be acidic.

Selected health-related aspects

A number of benefits can be ascribed to probiotic and prebiotic intake.[13,14] However, three areas of interest are described below.

Hypocholesterol action

The lipid hypothesis purports that dietary saturated fatty acids lead to an increase in blood cholesterol levels. This may have the effect of depositing cholesterol in the arterial wall, leading to atherosclerosis and possibly coronary heart disease. Some studies have hypothesised a role for the lactic microflora in systemically reducing blood lipid values.[15] However, this has not been unequivocally proven and there are contrasting data from human volunteer trials. Volunteer dietary trials should be carried out using a random double-blind placebo procedure, with unequivocal testing of bacterial changes and a range of human subjects.

Bowel cancer

In humans, colorectal cancer is thought to have a bacterial origin, with around 10 different carcinogens described that have been attributed to microbial events.[16] Dietary strategies that lead to a reduced accumulation of such products may be possible. First, dietary fibres and resistant starches may be fermented in the large gut to increase faecal bulk and reduce the residence time of such materials in the gut. Moreover, probiotics and prebiotics may modify the activities of enzymes that are involved in carcinogenesis, such as azoreductases, nitroreductases, β-glucuronidase, etc.

Effects on pathogens

The most compelling evidence for the success of probiotics and prebiotics probably lies in their ability to improve resistance to pathogens. Lactic acid excreting microorganisms are known for their inhibitory properties. In humans, viruses, protozoa, fungi and bacteria can all cause acute gastroenteritis. Viral infections play a major role, but bacteria are also of great significance.

There are a number of potential

mechanisms for probiotic microorganisms to reduce intestinal infections, both bacterial and viral.[1] First, metabolic end products such as acids excreted by these microorganisms may lower the gut pH to levels below those at which pathogens are able to compete effectively. Also, many lactobacilli and bifidobacterial species are able to excrete natural antibiotics, which can have a broad spectrum of activity. For the bifidobacteria, our studies have indicated that some species are able to exert antimicrobial effects on various Gram-positive and Gram-negative intestinal pathogens.[17] This includes the verocytotoxin strain of *Escherichia coli* 0157:H7 and campylobacters. Increased levels of bifidobacteria in the gut have the potential to improve resistance to infection.

Future developments

Prebiotics currently in use are modulators of gut function through their fermentation by groups such as bifidobacteria. However, it may be that improved functionality in the concept may be possible. This may include some of the following areas.

Increased persistence through the colon

One obvious attribute that an enhanced probiotic or prebiotic would possess is the ability to persist towards distal areas of the colon. Many common diseases of the human large bowel, such as ulcerative colitis and colonic cancer, arise in the left side. As such, enhanced functionality may arise in this part of the colon.

Anti-adhesive properties

An oligosaccharide with prebiotic properties may also have antiadhesive activities. This would add major functionality to the approach of altering gut pathogenesis. Binding of pathogens to these receptors is the first step in the colonisation process. There is much potential for developing prebiotics that incorporate such a receptor monosaccharide or oligosaccharide sequence. These molecules would thereby act as 'decoy' molecules for gut pathogens but also stimulate benign components of the microbiota. Such multifunctional prebiotics should increase host resistance to infection.

Attenuative properties

The prebiotic concept may be extrapolated further by considering an attenuation of virulence in certain food-borne pathogens. For example, the plant-derived carbohydrate cellobiose is able to repress the pathogenicity of *Listeria monocytogenes* through downregulation of its virulence factors.

Development of novel prebiotic food ingredients

At present, the most widespread use of a prebiotic is inulin, which is used as a dietary fibre, bulking agent and fat replacer in several foods. This is, however, a vastly underexplored area of research into prebiotics, and there is much potential for development of these oligosaccharides into other useful functional ingredients, such as sweeteners, surfactants, etc.

Synbiotics

One important development that is finding its way into functional foods is that of synbiotics. Here, a useful probiotic would be incorporated into an appropriate dietary vehicle with an appropriate prebiotic. The premise is that the selective substrate would be metabolised by the live addition in the gut. This would enhance probiotic survival, as well as offer the advantages of both gut microflora management techniques. A synbiotic has been defined as 'a mixture of probiotics and prebiotics that beneficially affects the host by improving the survival and implantation of live microbial dietary supplements in the gastrointestinal tract'. One example is a mixture of probiotic bifidobacteria with prebiotic fructo-oligosaccharides.

Encapsulation of probiotics with prebiotics

A further approach whereby probiotics could be targeted towards gut delivery would be to protect them through coating procedures. Encapsulation of the probiotic strains should protect them during passage through the stomach and small intestine. This approach could be extended with a view towards developing delivery systems that will release probiotic bacteria to the distal colon – a desirable outcome in terms of human health, as most large intestinal disorders arise in the left side. Prebiotics, which by definition enter the large intestine, could be used as the encapsulation material.

Species-level changes

Prebiotics currently act at the genus level, in that they induce group-level changes in bifidobacteria and/or lactobacilli. However, it may be that a more refined approach is necessary. For example, B. infantis is a more powerful inhibitor of pathogens than B. breve.[18] As such, it may be desirable to stimulate the former in certain circumstances. Reverse enzyme technology may be used to achieve this. In this context, we have generated galacto-oligosaccharides using lactase activities in certain probiotic bacteria. During fermentation studies these preferentially stimulate the strain from which they were derived.[19] This has hitherto been tested in pure culture. However, for a true prebiotic effect it is important that mixed culture studies are also carried out to confirm selectivity. The development of molecular-based procedures that allow high-fidelity discrimination of individual strains is required to facilitate this.

References

1. Gibson GR, Roberfroid MB, eds. *Colonic Microbiota, Nutrition and Health.* Dodrecht: Kluwer Academic, 1999.

2. Fuller R. Probiotics in man and animals. *J Appl Bacteriol* 1989; 66: 365–378.

3. Salminen S, Bouley C, Boutron-Ruault MC, *et al.* Functional food science and gastrointestinal physiology and function. *Br J Nutr* 1998; 80:S147–S171.

4. Collins MD, Gibson GR. Probiotics, prebiotics and synbiotics: Dietary approaches for the modulation of microbial ecology. *Am J Clin Nutr* 1999; 69:1052–1057.

5. Gibson GR, Roberfroid MB. Dietary modulation of the human colonic microbiota: introducing the concept of prebiotics. *J Nutr* 1995; 125:1401–1412.

6. McCartney AL, Gibson GR. The application of prebiotics in human health and nutrition. In: *Proceedings Lactic 97. Which Strains? For Which Products?* Adria Normandie, 1998: 59–73.

7. Wang X, Gibson GR. Effects of the in vitro fermentation of oligofructose and inulin by bacteria growing in the human large intestine. *J Appl Bacteriol* 1993; 75:373–380.

8. Williams C, Witherly SA, Buddington RK. Influence of dietary neosugar on selected bacterial groups of the human faecal microbiota. *Microb Ecology Health Dis* 1994; 7:91–97.

9. Kleessen B, Sykura B, Zunft H-J, Blaut M. Effects of inulin and lactose on fecal microflora, microbial activity and bowel habit in elderly constipated persons. *Am J Clin Nutr* 1997; 65:1397–1402.

10. Gibson GR, Beatty ER, Wang X, Cummings JH. Selective stimulation of bifidobacteria in the human colon by oligofructose and inulin. *Gastroenterology* 1995; 108:975–982.

11. Imamura L, Hisamitsu K, Kobashi K. Purification and characterization of β-fructofuranosidase from *Bifidobacterium infantis. Biol Pharmacol Bull* 1994; 17: 596–602.

12. Playne MJ, Crittenden R. Commercially available oligosaccharides. *Bull Int Dairy Foundation* 1996; 313:10–22.

13. Fuller R (ed). *Probiotics 2: Application and Practical Aspects.* Andover: Chapman and Hall, 1997.

14. Gibson GR, Macfarlane GT. Intestinal bacteria and disease. In: Gibson SAW, ed. *Human Health – the Contribution of Microorganisms.* London: Springer-Verlag, 1994: 53–62.

15. Gilliland SE, Nelson CR, Maxwell C. Assimilation of cholesterol by *Lactobacillus acidophilus. Appl Environ Microbiol* 1985; 49:377–381.

16. Reddy BS. Prevention of colon cancer by pre- and probiotics: evidence from laboratory studies. *Br J Nutr* 1998; 80:S219–S223.

17. Mackey BM, Gibson GR. *Escherichia coli*

0157 – from farm to fork and beyond. *Soc Gen Microbiol Q* 1997; 24:55–57.

18. Gibson GR, Wang X. Regulatory effects of bifidobacteria on the growth of other colonic bacteria. *J Appl Bacteriol* 1994; 77:412–420.

19. Rabui B, Jay AJ, Gibson GR, Rastall RA. Synthesis of novel galacto-oligosaccharides by β-galactosidases from *Bifidobacterium* and *Lactobacillus* species. *Appl Environ Microbiol* 2001 (in press).

Summary and observations

Glenn R Gibson

As the gut is the first point of contact for foods, the major influence on gastrointestinal function is diet. The availability of dietary residues is therefore a key determinant of gut physiology, affecting transit time and intestinal microbial function. This may have both negative and positive consequences for host health and welfare, with increasing interest being directed towards the role of gut processes in human nutrition.

These two chapters have examined two different aspects of the effect of food on gut health. First, the issue of food intolerance was described, using coeliac disease as a study model. Important correlations with food allergy, especially in infants, are described. The second chapter describes the role of gut bacteria in human health and overviews the use of prebiotic oligosaccharides in inducing a beneficial microbiota.

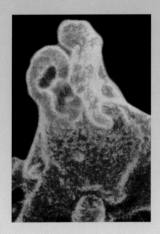

PART 4
Intestinal bacteria and mechanisms of disease

Genetically determined mucosal immune responses to normal resident luminal bacteria

10

R Balfour Sartor

The role of commensal bacteria in intestinal inflammation

Rodent models provide an extremely powerful tool to investigate the complex interplay of microbial, immunologic and neurohumoral mechanisms involved in the pathogenesis of chronic intestinal inflammation.[1-3] We have examined the hypothesis that chronic intestinal inflammation in genetically susceptible hosts is a result of an exaggerated cellular immune response to certain components of the predominantly anerobic bacterial population colonizing the distal ileum and colon. Inflammation is mediated by Th1 lymphocytes and macrophages, and genetic susceptibility is determined by a dysregulated immune response or a leaky mucosal barrier. The most compelling evidence supporting this hypothesis is the fact that in at least 11 separate animal models, intestinal inflammation fails to develop in the absence of luminal bacteria (Table 10.1).[4-6] This association of inflammation with luminal bacteria is universal in all of the studied genetically engineered rats and mice, and is seen in the vast majority of inducible models, with the only controversy being centered on the dextran sodium sulfate mouse model, which

Table 10.1
Animal models of colitis or enteritis in which intestinal inflammation is absent in the germ-free or sterile state

A. Mice: IL-2$^{-/-}$, IL-10 $^{-/-}$, TCRα $^{-/-}$, CD3ε transgenic, Samp-1/Yit, CD45RB^{hi} → SCID, DSS-induced
B. Rats: HLA B27 transgenic, indomethacin-induced
C. Guinea pigs: Carageenan-induced
D. Cottontop tamarin: Thiry–Vella loop

is not T-cell mediated in the most frequently studied acute phase.[7,8]

In the well-studied IL-10 knockout mouse model, germ-free mice have no evidence of histologic inflammation or weight loss and have normal mucosal levels of IL-12, interferon-γ (IFNγ) and IgG2a.[9] Within one week of colonization with specific pathogen-free (SPF) bacteria devoid of detectable intestinal *Helicobacter* species, IL-10 knockout mice develop histologic evidence of colitis with crypt hyperplasia, infiltration of mononuclear cells into the lamina propria, and loss of goblet cells. This colitis is most evident in the cecum and is progressive, reaching severe transmural inflammation with mucosal ulceration and a 50% mortality rate by 5 weeks of colonization. At this time, there is evidence of an aggressive Th1- and macrophage-mediated mucosal inflammatory response, with increased IL-12, IFNγ, IL-1β, TNF and IL-6. Interestingly, the age of a mouse at the time of bacterial colonization is important, as IL-10 knockout

mice colonized at birth with the same SPF organisms show only moderate inflammation confined to the mucosa at a similar age. Of considerable importance, wild-type mice of the same genetic background (129/C57 Bl6 mixture) exhibit no evidence of colitis or immune activation when colonized with the same organisms, confirming the non-pathogenic nature of these resident bacteria. In our hands, *Helicobacter hepaticus* does not influence activity of colitis in IL-10$^{-/-}$ mice, although Kullberg and colleagues[10,11] showed potentiation of colitis in IL-10$^{-/-}$ mice on an inbred C57/Bl6 background, which is a relatively resistant strain. CD4$^+$ mesenteric lymph node (MLN) cells isolated from SPF IL-10 knockout mice mount vigorous IFNγ responses when cultured with antigen-presenting cells pulsed overnight with lysates of homologous cecal bacteria, but wild-type mouse CD4$^+$ T cells show no increased IFNγ secretion over media controls. These results demonstrate that although resident bacteria are required for the induction of immune-mediated chronic intestinal inflammation, host genetic background is a key factor determining susceptibility to this inflammatory response.

Mechanisms of T-cell activation

The finding that T lymphocytes mediate chronic inflammation in these rodent models led us to investigate the mechanisms by which luminal bacteria activate mucosal T cells in the CD3ϵ_{26} transgenic mouse model. These mice lack T lymphocytes and natural killer cells, have an atrophic thymus, and develop colitis within 4–6 weeks after bone marrow transplantation from a wild-type murine donor or within 2–4 weeks after receiving MLN cells isolated from Tgϵ_{26} mice with colitis.[12] In collaboration with Cox Terhorst, we performed a series of experiments in which germ-free or SPF Tgϵ_{26} mice received either bone marrow transplant from normal mice, or MLN transfer from either SPF Tgϵ_{26} mice with colitis or germ-free Tgϵ_{26} mice after bone marrow transplant.[13] In each situation, SPF recipients developed Th1-mediated colitis but germ-free recipients had no clinical, histologic or immunologic evidence of intestinal inflammation. Of considerable importance, germ-free Tgϵ_{26} transgenic recipients of a bone marrow transplant develop active colitis within 2–4 weeks after being moved to an SPF environment, and MLN cells from germ-free mice transferred disease to SPF immunodeficient recipients. The presence of functional mucosal T cells in the germ-free mice was demonstrated by near-equal stimulation of intracytoplasmic IFNγ and TNF in CD4$^+$ MLN cells isolated from germ-free SPF ϵ_{26} transgenic mice after bone marrow transplant with anti-CD3 antibody. Furthermore, CD4$^+$ MLN cells from SPF ϵ_{26} mice following bone marrow transplant had vigorous IFNγ responses to cecal bacterial lysates from SPF mice, but no response to germ-free cecal contents or to lysates of colonic epithelial cells isolated from germ-free mice. These results demonstrate that resident luminal bacteria are required for immune activation and colitis, continuous bacterial stimulation is necessary to sustain colitis even after T cells are activated, and autoimmune responses are not observed in this model.

Differential effects of bacterial species

The HLA B27 transgenic rat model was used to demonstrate that different resident luminal bacterial species have variable capacities to induce inflammation in genetically susceptible hosts. As in the IL-10 knockout mouse, B27 transgenic rats do not develop colitis, arthritis or gastritis in the sterile environment, but Th1-mediated colitis with extraintestinal inflammation develops within 1 month of bacterial colonization.[14,15] Studies with defined bacterial populations implicated *Bacteroides vulgatus* as a key strain capable of inducing colitis and mucosal immune cell activation.[15] This observation was confirmed by monoassociation with *B. vulgatus*, with no inflammation developing in the littermates colonized with *Escherichia coli*.[16] Protective effects with *Lactobacillus* GG indicate the potential for protective effects by certain luminal constituents.[17] However, *B. vulgatus* does not universally induce colitis, as only minimal inflammation is observed in gnotobiotic IL-10 knockout and $Tg\varepsilon_{26}$ transgenic mice colonized with this organism. However, we very recently demonstrated that IL-10$^{-/-}$ mice monoassociated with a human oral Enterococcus faecalis isolate develop aggressive distal colitis, with increased mucosal IL-12 expression and enhanced secretion of IFNγ from MLN cells stimulated with anti-CD3.[18] This inflammation has a histologic appearance of crypt hyperplasia, goblet cell depletion and mononuclear cell infiltration in the lamina propria similar to SPF IL-10 knockout mice, but differs from the SPF mice in that *E. faecalis*-induced colitis is distal, whereas germ-free IL-10$^{-/-}$ mice colonized with SPF bacteria have a predominantly cecal inflammatory response.[9] MLN CD4$^+$ T cells from the *E. faecalis*-monoassociated mice produce abundant IFNγ in response to *E. faecalis* lysates but not with *E. coli* lysates. Of greater physiologic importance, MLN CD4$^+$ cells from SPF IL-10 knockout mice exhibit vigorous IFNg secretion to *E. faecalis* lysates. Together, these results indicate that certain bacterial species have preferential abilities to induce Th1-mediated colitis. Of considerable potential clinical relevance, the host genetic background appears to determine mucosal T-cell responses to individual luminal resident bacterial species. It is quite possible that each genetically defined subset of Crohn's disease and ulcerative colitis may have a different dominant microbial stimulus.

Dysbiosis

In very preliminary observations we have raised the possibility of a varied composition of resident bacteria in rats and mice with colitis versus those without colitis. In both the IL-10 knockout and HLA B27 transgenic models, cecal lysates from animals with colitis induced more vigorous T-cell responses than were seen from identically prepared lysates of cecal contents from rodents without colitis. Whether these results are caused by an expansion of immunogenic bacterial species, selective diminution of protective bacterial constituents, induction of virulence factors in commensal bacteria by the inflammatory milieu, or the presence of immunologically active cytokines of host origin in the cecal lysates remains to be determined.

Induction of protective responses in normal hosts

From parallel studies it is now evident that resident luminal bacteria are also capable of inducing protective (regulatory) immunologic responses in genetically resistant (normal) hosts. Key cytokines involved in these tolerogenic responses are IL-10 and TGFβ, which exert immunosuppressive activities. In elegant co-transfer studies, Cong and Elson[19,20] showed the ability of bacterial antigen-specific T$_{R1}$ lymphocytes to prevent the transfer of colitis by bacterial responsive

Th1 lymphocytes in immunodeficient (SCID) mouse recipients. *In vitro* studies with splenic and MLN cells isolated from IL-10 knockout mice versus wild-type controls demonstrate dose- and time-dependent enhanced IL-12, IFNγ and TNF secretion in response to LPS stimulation in the absence of endogenous IL-10.[21] This increased proinflammatory cytokine production was not dependent on the presence of colitis, as similar trends were seen in cells from germ-free IL-10 knockout mice with no clinical or histologic evidence of colitis. Wild-type mouse cells produce IL-10 in response to LPS, although peak responses were delayed, being seen at 72 hours post LPS stimulation. Similar results were seen in MLN cells from HLA B27 transgenic rats stimulated *in vitro* with cecal lysates. Compared with wild-type controls, B27 transgenic rats had significant elevations of IL-12 and IFNγ, but decreased secretion of IL-10 after stimulation with cecal lysates. The ratio of IL-10 to IL-12 was between four and nine times higher in wild type mice. Somewhat surprisingly, T-cell depletion studies showed that the majority of IL-10 was produced by non-T-cell populations with B lymphocytes showing the greatest degree of intracytoplasmic staining.

Conclusions

In summary, these studies clearly indicate that resident intestinal bacteria profoundly influence the mucosal and systemic immune response. Homeostasis vs. chronic intestinal inflammation is determined by the host's genetically determined immunologic response to the luminal microenvironment. Normal, genetically resistant animals with regulated immunologic responses develop tolerance mediated by regulatory T cells and dendritic cells/macrophages which secrete IL-10, TGFβ and protective prostaglandins. At the opposite extreme, susceptible hosts with genetically dysregulated immune responses develop chronic relapsing intestinal inflammation mediated by macrophages and Th1 lymphocytes which secrete a proinflammatory profile of cytokines and eicosanoids. Animal models can be profitably used to further dissect dominant microbial stimuli of intestinal inflammation, to explore the mechanisms of dysbiosis in colitic animals, and to determine novel means of reversing the ability of luminal bacteria to induce pathogenic immune responses. It is this author's bias that simultaneous elimination of the detrimental components of the resident luminal bacteria, expanding the beneficial microbial population, paralyzing the pathogenic immune response and facilitating healing of the mucosal barrier, will afford the best chance to change the natural history of these chronic spontaneously relapsing disorders.

References

1. Fiocchi C. Inflammatory bowel disease: etiology and pathogenesis. *Gastroenterology* 1998; 115:182–205.

2. Sartor RB. Pathogenesis and immune mechanisms of chronic inflammatory bowel diseases. *Am J Gastroenterol* 1997; 92:5S–11S.

3. Strober W, Ludviksson BR, Fuss IJ. The pathogenesis of mucosal inflammation in murine models of inflammatory bowel disease and Crohn's disease. *Ann Intern Med* 1998; 128:848–856.

4. Sartor RB. Microbial factors in the pathogenesis of Crohn's disease, ulcerative colitis and experimental intestinal inflammation. In: Kirsner JB, ed. *Inflammatory Bowel Diseases* 5th edn. Philadelphia: WB Saunders, 1999: 153–178.

5. Sartor RB, Veltkamp C. Interactions between enteric bacteria and the immune system which determine mucosal homeostasis vs. chronic intestinal inflammation: lessons from rodent models. In: Rogler G, Kullmann F, Rutgeerts P, Sartor RB, Scholmerich J, eds. IBD at the End of Its First Century. *Proceedings of the Falk Symposium 111.* Dordrecht: Kluwer Academic, 2000: 30–41.

6. Sartor RB. Intestinal microflora in human and experimental inflammatory bowel disease. *Curr Opin Gastroenterol* 2001; 17:324–330.

7. Axelsson LG, Midtvedt T, Bylund-Fellenius AC. The role of intestinal bacteria, bacterial translocation and endotoxin in dextran sodium sulphate-induced colitis in the mouse. *Microb Ecol Health Dis* 1996; 9:225–237.

8. Tlaskalova H, Stepankova R, Hudcovic T, *et al.* The role of bacterial microflora in development of dextran sodium sulphate (DSS) induced colitis in immunocompetent

and immunodeficient mice. *Microb Ecol Health Dis* 1999; 11:115–116.

9. Sellon RK, Tonkonogy S, Schultz M, *et al.* Resident enteric bacteria are necessary for development of spontaneous colitis and immune system activation in interleukin-10-deficient mice. *Infect Immun* 1998; 66: 5224–5231.

10. Dieleman LA, Arends A, Tonkonogy SL, *et al.* *Helicobacter hepaticus* does not induce or potentiate colitis in interleukin-10-deficient mice. *Infect Immun* 2000; 68:5107–5113.

11. Kullberg MC, Ward JM, Gorelick P, *et al.* *Helicobacter hepaticus* triggers colitis in specific-pathogen-free interleukin-10 (IL-10)-deficient mice through an IL-12 and gamma interferon-dependent mechanism. *Infect Immun* 1998; 66:5157–5166.

12. Hollander GA, Simpson SJ, Mizoguchi E, *et al.* Severe colitis in mice with aberrant thymic selection. *Immunity* 1995; 3:27–38.

13. Veltkamp C, Tonkonogy SL, de Yong Y, *et al.* Continuous stimulation by normal luminal bacteria is essential for the development and perpetuation of colitis in TG epsilon 26 mice after bone marrow transplantation or adoptive transfer. *Gastroenterology* 2001; 120:900–913

14. Taurog JD, Richardson JA, Croft JT, *et al.* The germfree state prevents development of gut and joint inflammatory disease in HLA-B27 transgenic rats. *J Exp Med* 1994; 180:2359–2364.

15. Rath HC, Herfarth HH, Ikeda JS, *et al.* Normal luminal bacteria, especially Bacteroides species, mediate chronic colitis, gastritis, and arthritis in HLA-B27/human beta2 microglobulin transgenic rats. *J Clin Invest* 1996; 98:945–953.

16. Rath HC, Wilson KH, Sartor RB. Differential induction of colitis and gastritis in HLA-B27

transgenic rats selectively colonized with *Bacteroides vulgatus* and *Escherichia coli*. *Infect Immun* 1999; 67:2969–2974.

17. Dieleman LA, Goerres M, Arends A, Springer TA, Sartor RB. *Lactobacillus* GG prevents recurrence of colitis in HLA B$_{27}$ transgenic rats after antibiotic treatment. *Gastroenterology* 2000; 118:A814 (Abstract).

18. Kim SC, Tonkonogy SL, Balish E, Brackett DR, Warner T, Sartor RB. IL-10 deficient mice monoassociated with nonpathogenic *Enterococcus faecalis* develop chronic colitis. *Gastroenterology* 2001; 120:A82.

19. Cong Y, Brandwein SL, McCabe RP, *et al*. CD4+ T cells reactive to enteric bacterial antigens in spontaneously colitic C3H/HeJBir mice: increased T helper cell type 1 response and ability to transfer disease. *J Exp Med* 1998; 187:855–864.

20. Cong Y, Weaver CT, Lazenby A, Sundberg JP, Elson CO. T-regulatory-1 (TR1) cells prevent colitis induced by enteric bacterial antigen-reactive pathogenic TH1 cells. *Gastroenterology* 2000; 118:A683 (Abstract).

21. Kim S, Tonkonogy SL, Sartor RB. Role of endogenous IL-10 in downregulating proinflammatory cytokine expression. *Gastroenterology* 2001; 120:A183 (Abstract).

22. Tonkonogy SL, Hoentjen F, Sprengers D, Goerres M, Sartor RB, Dieleman LA. Altered profile of the immunoregulatory cytokines IL-10, IL-12 and IFN-gamma in HLA B27 transgenic rat mesenteric lymph node cells stimulated with cecal bacterial components. *FASEB J* 2001; 15:A372 (Abstract).

Defensins and antimicrobial peptides

Ailsa L Hart

11

Introduction

With regard to host defence, the gastrointestinal tract is faced
with many challenges. The mucosal immune system is poised
to sense the local environment, and the critical design
paradox is that it needs to avoid potentially harmful responses
to dietary antigens and the commensal flora while responding
rapidly to episodic challenges from pathogens. The healthy
individual's response to the normal flora is not due to the
non-immunogenicity of the flora, but rather to a highly
regulated response. From a teleological viewpoint this
response can be seen as a direct consequence of the immune
system's need to recognise and respond to pathogens. There is
a constant level of highly regulated physiological
inflammation in operation, involving a network of
connectivity between the enteric flora, the innate and
adaptive mucosal immune systems, neurons, muscles,
fibroblasts, endothelial cells and epithelial cells.

In particular, innate immune defences include the
production of defensins, a group of endogenous antimicrobial
peptides, interest in which continues for several reasons.
These peptides are adapted to contribute to mucosal barrier

function in the hostile environment of the intestinal lumen. Knowledge of their structure, function and altered expression in various disease states, including chronic inflammation, will provide a greater understanding of their role in this environment. They may prove to be useful as templates for new 'antibiotics' or 'immunostimulants'.

Antimicrobial peptides

Antimicrobial peptides are part of an ancient immunological system. Hundreds have been found in plants and animals, from molluscs to humans. As a class, the peptides are diverse and range from linear α-helical molecules to disulphide-bonded, β-sheet containing peptides.[1] Despite differences in their primary and secondary structures, these peptides have antimicrobial activity against a broad range of microbes at micromolar concentrations. They are usually cationic, with spatially separated hydrophobic and charged regions. This arrangement allows them to insert into phospholipid membranes and form pores. They have a greater affinity for disrupting microbial membranes rich in anionic phospholipids than host cell membranes that contain neutral phospholipids and in this way the host cells may be protected from concomitant damage. Other proposed mechanisms of microbicidal activity include disruption of bacterial energy metabolism

and interference with biosynthetic pathways.

Defensins

In mammals, defensins are one of the major families of antimicrobial peptides. Depending on the specific pattern of their cysteine spacing and disulphide connections, defensins fall into different structural classes: α, β, and the recently defined θ class. Although the disulphide linkages of the α and β defensins differ, their three-dimensional structures are similar,[2] and their genes reside in the same gene cluster on the short arm of chromosome 8 (8p23), indicating a common evolutionary origin.[3–5]

The α-defensins were among the first antimicrobial peptides to be discovered and are the major constituents of primary granules of neutrophils.[6,7] In humans, the α-defensins, termed human neutrophil peptides (HNP)-1–4, account for about 5% of the total cellular protein of neutrophils. Other α-defensins are abundantly expressed in Paneth cells at the base of the crypts of Lieberkühn in the small intestine.[8,9]

The β-defensins were discovered in the airway epithelial cells of cattle, but have since been found in epithelial cells of the human skin, kidneys and gastrointestinal tract.[10] Human intestinal epithelial cells constitutively produce human β-defensin (HBD)-1, whereas other human β-defensins, for example HBD-

2, are inducibly upregulated in response to epithelial cell infection or stimulation of epithelial cells with proinflammatory cytokines.[11,12] Moreover, HBD-2 functions as an NF-κB target gene in the intestinal epithelium, as blocking NF-κB activation inhibits the upregulated expression of HBD-2 in response to bacterial infection or stimulation with cytokines. In addition, a novel human β-defensin 3 (HBD-3) has been found in human colonic tissue and appears to be preferentially expressed in patients with ulcerative colitis.[13] Human β-defensins appear to play a role in alerting the adaptive immune system. HBD-1 and HBD-2 have been shown to be involved in attracting both immature dendritic cells and memory T cells *in vitro*, which initiate a primary and a recall immune response, respectively.[14] The effect was mediated by the CCR6 chemokine receptor because β-defensins effectively competed with the receptor's ligand macrophage inflammatory protein-3α (MIP-3α). If this mechanism functions *in vivo*, the release of these defensins could recruit dendritic cells and memory T cells to infected tissues, thereby promoting the development of adaptive immunity.

The θ-defensin was recently isolated from rhesus macaque neutrophils.[15] This novel molecule appears to be generated by head-to-tail splicing of the products of two similarly truncated α-defensin genes. Although otherwise similar to α-defensins with six

cysteines, these defensin genes contained a 'premature' stop codon, resulting in the generation of two abbreviated defensin molecules that each donated nine amino acids to the final 18 amino acid cyclic product – a θ-defensin stabilised by three parallel disulphide bonds. This conformation enables the molecule to have full antimicrobial activity at salt concentrations present in blood, a feature not shared by the acyclic form, which makes them interesting candidates for development as antibiotics.

Defensins in Paneth cells

Paneth cells populate the crypts of Lieberkühn in the small intestine and became implicated as effectors of mucosal barrier function when lysozyme and secretory phospholipase A_2,[16,17] in addition to defensins, were found in these cells. All of these molecules have antimicrobial properties, and there may be a synergism between them. However, despite the association of these cells with innate immune function, fully differentiated Paneth cells develop in germ-free rodents and when fetal human tissue is implanted under subcutaneous skin flaps,[18,19] implying that luminal bacteria and dietary factors are not crucial to the development of this lineage.

In mice, biochemical and genetic studies have revealed that there are at least 20 crypt α-defensins (termed cryptdins) in a single crypt of Lieberkühn,[20] whereas in humans two

Paneth cell α-defensins have been identified, human defensin (HD)-5 and HD-6.[21] These peptides are differentially expressed along the longitudinal axis of the small intestine, with increasing abundance distally, but they are not detected in the colon. Cryptidin genes are active in the intestinal epithelium prior to Paneth cell differentiation, indicating that these defensins are early markers of crypt ontogeny. Intraluminal bacteria, lipopolysaccharide, lipoteichoic acid, lipid A and muramyl dipeptide, but not live fungi and protozoa, can stimulate Paneth cell secretion, although the specific antigens are unknown.[22] In addition, cholinergic agonists cause Paneth cell degranulation, which is inhibited by atropine, a muscarinic antagonist, indicating a role for cholinergic enteric nerves in the mechanism.[16,23]

As a family, α-defensins have a range of activity against Gram-positive and Gram-negative bacteria, fungi, spirochaetes, protozoa and envelope viruses. Under optimised conditions, minimum bactericidal concentrations are observed at 1–2μM. Recombinant human Paneth cell defensin, HD-5, is active against *Listeria monocytogenes, Escherichia coli, Salmonella typhimurium* and *Candida albicans*.[24] The recombinant HD-5 peptide retains activity even in the presence of physiological concentrations of trypsin, evidence that this peptide could function within the hostile environment of the intestinal lumen. More extensive

structure–function studies have been possible with the mouse Paneth cell α-defensins. Of these, cryptidin-4 is the most cationic and has the greatest antimicrobial activity.[20] Mouse cryptidins 1, 2, 3 and 6 differ from each other only by one to four amino acids, yet they have been shown to exhibit a high degree of specificity against certain target microorganisms. Subtle changes in the primary structure of these molecules are important for their biological activity. Thus, intestinal Paneth cells contribute to innate immunity by sensing bacteria and bacterial antigens, and are able to discharge microbicidal peptides at effective concentrations.[22,25]

Post-translational processing of the amino terminus of the defensin molecule may affect its antimicrobial activity. Recent studies have shown that the post-translational processing of cryptidin precursors is dependent on the proteolytic activity of matrilysin (matrix metalloprotease 7) and occurs primarily intracellularly. Matrilysin-null mice lack mature cryptidins, and their Paneth cells accumulate unprocessed cryptidins. Although matrilysin-null mice have an apparently normal phenotype, they are defective in their ability to clear orally administered *Salmonella typhimurium*, providing evidence for the role of mature defensins in controlling bacterial colonisation in the small intestine.[26]

Neutrophil α-defensins have a variety of non-microbicidal activities, leading to speculation that Paneth cell α-defensins may also exhibit more diverse functions. Some neutrophil α-defensins have been reported:

- to be chemotactic for monocytes and T lymphocytes;
- to be mitogenic;
- to inhibit *in vitro* natural killer cell activity;
- to inhibit corticosteroid biosynthesis;
- to alter epithelial barrier integrity in cultured cells;
- to be cytotoxic to mammalian cells under certain circumstances.

Evidence that the mouse cryptidin peptides may be multifunctional was shown by the fact that cryptidins-2 or -3 stimulate chloride secretion by forming anion-conductive channels when administered apically to T84 cells, a human intestinal epithelial cell line.[27] If Paneth cell α-defensins elicit chloride secretion *in situ*, the peptides could contribute to a paracrine mechanism that clears the crypt lumen and distributes granule constituents to villous surfaces.

Defensins and inflammatory bowel disease

With regard to inflammatory bowel disease, the aetiology appears to involve three interacting elements:

- genetic susceptibility;

- priming by an environmental factor, which appears to be part of the normal enteric flora;
- immune-mediated tissue injury.

The genetic susceptibility may determine the dysregulated immune response, a leaky mucosal barrier, an imbalance in the enteric flora,[28] or a combination of these. It is not clear whether the barrier function is primarily compromised by intrinsic defects in epithelial integrity, by infection with pathogens, or by loss or changes in commensal-dependent signals necessary to maintain it. A defect in defensin expression or function may contribute to barrier dysfunction and subsequent inflammation. Alternatively, it is theoretically possible that the barrier function could be enhanced by such molecules. It has been noted that there is altered expression of defensins in inflammatory bowel disease. For example, alterations have been found in HNP 1–3,[29] HD-2[30] and HD-5 and 6 expression.[31] It is recognised that Paneth cell metaplasia occurs in the colon of patients with ulcerative colitis,[25,32] but the functional characteristics of these cells remains unclear. It is suggested that these cells do secrete antimicrobial granules in response to bacterial stimuli, indicating a possible protective role in inflamed tissue,[33] and it has been shown recently that HD-5 is expressed by metaplastic Paneth cells in the colon in Crohn's disease.[34] DNA microarrays have been used to examine global gene expression profiles of inflamed colonic tissue, and the natural antimicrobial defensin DEFA5 and DEFA6 genes have been shown to be particularly overexpressed in Crohn's disease.[35]

In summary, improving our understanding of Paneth cell biology and their antimicrobial peptides may help to clarify the molecular interactions in the crypt microenvironment. It will be interesting to assess the role of defensins in health and disease states, such as inflammatory bowel disease. The structure–function relationships, biological activities and regulation of the Paneth cell defensins offer promise as areas of future research. In particular, their role in innate host defence mechanisms, with the possible link to adaptive immune systems, may lead to therapeutic strategies that enhance the host defence.

References

1. Boman HG. Peptide antibiotics and their role in innate immunity. *Annu Rev Immunol* 1995; 13:61–92.

2. White SH, Wimley WC, Selsted ME. Structure, function, and membrane integration of defensins. *Curr Opin Struct Biol* 1995; 5:521–527.

3. Harder J, Siebert R, Zhang Y, *et al.* Mapping of the gene encoding human beta-defensin-2 (DEFB2) to chromosome region 8p22-p23.1. *Genomics* 1997; 46:472–475.

4. Liu L, Zhao C, Heng HH, Ganz T. The human beta-defensin-1 and alpha-defensins are encoded by adjacent genes: two peptide families with differing disulfide topology share a common ancestry. *Genomics* 1997; 43: 316–320.

5. Sparkes RS, Kronenberg M, Heinzmann C, Daher KA, Klisak I, Ganz T *et al.* Assignment of defensin gene(s) to human chromosome 8p23. *Genomics* 1989; 5:240–244.

6. Ganz T, Selsted ME, Szklarek D, *et al.* Defensins. Natural peptide antibiotics of human neutrophils. *J Clin Invest* 1985; 76:1427–1435.

7. Selsted ME, Harwig SS, Ganz T, Schilling JW, Lehrer RI. Primary structures of three human neutrophil defensins. *J Clin Invest* 1985; 76:1436–1439.

8. Selsted ME, Miller SI, Henschen AH, Ouellette AJ. Enteric defensins: antibiotic peptide components of intestinal host defense. *J Cell Biol* 1992; 118:929–936.

9. Harwig SS, Eisenhauer PB, Chen NP, Lehrer RI. Cryptdins: endogenous antibiotic peptides of small intestinal Paneth cells. *Adv Exp Med Biol* 1995; 371A:251–255.

10. Diamond G, Bevins CL. beta-Defensins: endogenous antibiotics of the innate host defense response. *Clin Immunol Immunopathol* 1998; 88:221–225.

11. O'Neil DA, Porter EM, Elewaut D, *et al.* Expression and regulation of the human beta-defensins hBD-1 and hBD-2 in intestinal epithelium. *J Immunol* 1999; 163:6718–6724.

12. O'Neil DA, Cole SP, Martin-Porter E, *et al.* Regulation of human beta-defensins by gastric epithelial cells in response to infection with *Helicobacter pylori* or stimulation with interleukin-1. *Infect Immun* 2000; 68: 5412–5415.

13. Wehkamp J, Harder J, Herrlinger KR, *et al.*

Human b-defensin 3: A novel antimicrobial peptide preferentially expressed in ulcerative colitis. *Gastroenterology* 2001; 120(Suppl 1): 962 (Abstract).

14. Yang D, Chertov O, Bykovskaia SN, Chen Q, Buffo MJ, Shogan J *et al.* Beta-defensins: linking innate and adaptive immunity through dendritic and T cell CCR6. *Science* 1999; 286:525–528.

15. Tang YQ, Yuan J, Osapay G, *et al.* A cyclic antimicrobial peptide produced in primate leukocytes by the ligation of two truncated alpha-defensins. *Science* 1999; 286:498–502.

16. Peeters T, Vantrappen G. The Paneth cell: a source of intestinal lysozyme. *Gut* 1975; 16:553–558.

17. Harwig SS, Tan L, Qu XD, Cho Y, Eisenhauer PB, Lehrer RI. Bactericidal properties of murine intestinal phospholipase A2. *J Clin Invest* 1995; 95:603–610.

18. Rubin DC, Roth KA, Birkenmeier EH, Gordon JI. Epithelial cell differentiation in normal and transgenic mouse intestinal isografts. *J Cell Biol* 1991; 113:1183–1192.

19. Winter HS, Hendren RB, Fox CH, *et al.* Human intestine matures as nude mouse xenograft. *Gastroenterology* 1991; 100:89–98.

20. Ouellette AJ, Hsieh MM, Nosek MT, *et al.* Mouse Paneth cell defensins: primary structures and antibacterial activities of numerous cryptdin isoforms. *Infect Immun* 1994; 62:5040–5047.

21. Mallow EB, Harris A, Salzman N, *et al.* Human enteric defensins. Gene structure and developmental expression. *J Biol Chem* 1996; 271:4038–4045.

22. Ayabe T, Satchell DP, Wilson CL, Parks WC, Selsted ME, Ouellette AJ. Secretion of microbicidal alpha-defensins by intestinal Paneth cells in response to bacteria. *Nat Immunol* 2000; 1:113–118.

23. Satoh Y. Atropine inhibits the degranulation of Paneth cells in ex-germ-free mice. *Cell Tissue Res* 1988; 253:397–402.

24. Porter EM, van Dam E, Valore EV, Ganz T. Broad-spectrum antimicrobial activity of human intestinal defensin 5. *Infect Immun* 1997; 65:2396–2401.

25. Stamp GW, Poulsom R, Chung LP, *et al.* Lysozyme gene expression in inflammatory bowel disease. *Gastroenterology* 1992; 103: 532–538.

26. Wilson CL, Ouellette AJ, Satchell DP, *et al.* Regulation of intestinal alpha-defensin activation by the metalloproteinase matrilysin in innate host defense. *Science* 1999; 286: 113–117.

27. Lencer WI, Cheung G, Strohmeier GR, *et al.* Induction of epithelial chloride secretion by channel-forming cryptdins 2 and 3. *Proc Natl Acad Sci USA* 1997; 94:8585–8589.

28. Van de Merwe JP, Stegeman JH, Hazenberg MP. The resident faecal flora is determined by genetic characteristics of the host. Implications for Crohn's disease? *Antonie Van Leeuwenhoek* 1983; 49:119–124.

29. de Weerth A, Reiser AC, Bisker M, *et al.* Overexpression of human neutrophil peptides in gastrointestinal tissues of patients with active inflammatory bowel disease. *Gastroenterology* 2001; 120(Suppl 1):1906 (Abstract).

30. Wehkamp J, Fellerman K, Herrlinger KR, *et al.* Human beta defensin 2 is induced in ulcerative colitis but not in Crohn's disease. *Gastroenterology* 2000: 118(Suppl 2):1898 (Abstract).

31. Wehkamp J, Fellerman K, Herrlinger KR, Baxman S, Rudolph B, Stange. Intestinal mRNA expression of human defensins in inflammatory bowel disease. *Gastroenterology* 1999; 116:G4114 (Abstract).

32. Sommers SC. Mast cells and Paneth cells in ulcerative colitis. *Gastroenterology* 1966; 51: 841–850.

33. Ayabe T, Maemoto A, Ashida T, *et al.* Functional studies of colonic Paneth cells in patients with ulcerative colitis. *Gastroenterology* 2001; 120(Suppl 1):2668 (Abstract).

34. Cunliffe RN, Rose FR, Keyte J, Abberley L, Chan WC, Mahida YR. Human defensin 5 is stored in precursor form in normal Paneth cells and is expressed by some villous epithelial cells and by metaplastic Paneth cells in the colon in inflammatory bowel disease. *Gut* 2001; 48:176–185.

35. Lawrance IC, Fiocchi C, Chakravarti S. Ulcerative colitis and Crohn's disease: distinctive gene expression profiles and novel susceptibility candidate genes. *Hum Mol Genet* 2001; 10:445–456.

Defending against enteric infections

Martin F Kagnoff

12

Introduction

The mucosa that lines the human colon and small intestine is a site of chronic regulated 'physiologic' inflammation (Figure 12.1). This contrasts markedly with other mucosal sites and

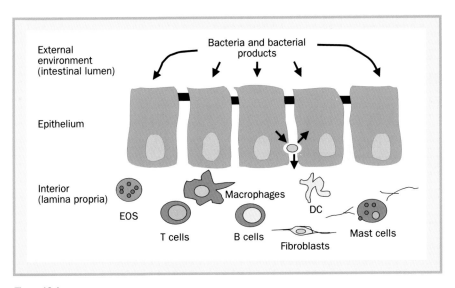

Figure 12.1
The intestinal mucosa is 'physiologically inflamed'.

the skin. Thus, if the numbers of T and B lymphocytes, eosinophils, mast cells, macrophages and dendritic cells that are present in the human intestinal tract were to be present in other sites, those sites would be considered to be sites of chronic pathological inflammation. This chapter focuses on the role of the intestinal epithelium in defending against enteric infections, with an emphasis on work by several different investigators during their stay in the Laboratory of Mucosal Immunology at the University of California, San Diego. The reader should also note that many scientists have contributed new information to this field, but could not be referenced because of the brevity of this chapter.

Intestinal epithelial cells as an integral component of the mucosal immune system

The intestinal mucosa is lined by a single layer of epithelial cells that separates the host's internal milieu from the intestinal lumen and the external environment. These cells are an initial site of cellular interaction between the host and the luminal contents. Thus, the epithelium must function to maintain an adequate barrier to luminal contents, while concurrently mediating absorptive and secretory functions that are essential to host survival. The epithelial layer uses a number of strategies to ensure that it functions as an

effective barrier to protect the host from the enormous universe of antigenic material from ingested foods, as well as bacteria and bacterial products, the latter being most prevalent in humans in the colon and distal small intestine.

In addition to interactions with the normal commensal microbial flora in the intestinal tract, the intestinal mucosa from time to time encounters enteropathogenic microbes. These pathogens may simply interact with the apical membrane of epithelial cells, may frankly invade epithelial cells or, alternatively, pass between epithelial cells, perhaps aided by dendritic cells,[1] or enter the host through specialized cells overlying mucosal lymphoid follicles, termed M cells.[2,3] Infected epithelial cells may ultimately undergo cytolysis or death by apoptosis.[4] Various enteric pathogens have developed strategies to alter these latter cellular processes e.g. *Cryptosporidium parvum* can inhibit epithelial cell apoptosis, and this is likely to be a strategy to prolong its survival in epithelial cells.[5,6]

The intestinal epithelium is now known to function as a central relay system and signal integrator in a complex communications network that transmits signals from luminal commensal microbes, microbial products and pathogenic bacteria to cells in the underlying lamina propria. Moreover, consistent with the role of the intestinal epithelial cells as an integral component of the mucosal immune system, epithelial cells constitutively express or can be induced to express receptors and products important for host mucosal and acquired immunity. These include, for example, cytokine receptors (e.g. putative receptors for IL-1, IL-4, IL-6, IL-7, IL-9, IL-10, IL-15, IL-17, IFN-γ, GM-CSF and TNFα),[7–15] receptors for several chemokines (e.g. CXCR4, CCR5, CCR6, CX3CR1),[16–18] Toll-like receptors,[19] MHC class II molecules and non-classic MHC class I molecules (e.g. CD1d, MICA)[20,21] (Figure 12.2).

Intestinal epithelial cells also can be induced to upregulate the *NOS2* gene in response to bacterial infection or stimulation with proinflammatory cytokines, which is accompanied by increased epithelial cell production of nitric oxide (NO),[22] and upregulate the gene that encodes for the inducible isoform of cyclo-oxygenase, cyclo-oxygenase (COX)-2, which can result in increased epithelial cell production of

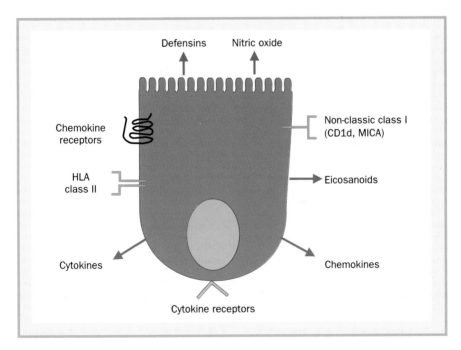

Figure 12.2
Intestinal epithelial cells are an integral component of the mucosal immune system.

prostaglandins, most notably PGE_2.[23] NO has an array of antimicrobial activities, whereas PGE_2 can act in an autocrine/paracrine manner to alter epithelial cell secretory processes important in the host response to microbial infection. Moreover, human intestinal epithelial cells constitutively produce known anti-microbial peptides, including human β-defensin (HBD)-1 and other human β-defensins (e.g. HBD-2) are inducibly upregulated in response to epithelial cell infection or stimulation of epithelial cells with proinflammatory cytokines.[24,25] Although this chapter focuses on the role of the epithelium in signaling and regulating the onset of the host mucosal response to infection, it should be noted that epithelial cells cannot be viewed in isolation and that cells in the lamina propria also signal and communicate with each other, as well as with the epithelium, through the release of mediators and via signals delivered by the enteric nervous system.

Role of intestinal epithelium in defending against enteric pathogens

We have successfully used enteropathogenic microbial agents to probe the repertoire of human epithelial cell responses that may be important in host–microbial interactions and cross-talk, especially with respect to host

mucosal innate and acquired immunity.[26] In this regard, we have taken advantage of microbial pathogens that are non-invasive for human intestinal epithelial cells,[27] those that enter epithelial cells but maintain an intraepithelial lifestyle and do not invade deeper into the mucosal or systemically,[5,28–31] and those that are frankly invasive in the host.[4,22–24,32–39] Examples of non-invasive pathogens include the protozoan parasite *Giardia lamblia* and pathogenic non-invasive strains of *E. coli*. Both of these pathogens engage in cross-talk with the human epithelium but induce host responses of a very different nature. The response to *Giardia* involves mainly mechanisms important for intraluminal host defense (e.g. IgA, competition for arginine, a precursor of nitric oxide).[27] In contrast, the response to pathogenic non-invasive strains of *Escherichia coli* involves both mucosal inflammation and intraluminal defense.[40,41] Examples of microbial pathogens that we have used to explore epithelial cell responses to intraepithelial cell pathogens include *C. parvum* and *Chlamydia trachomatis*,[28–31] whereas *Salmonella*, *Shigella*, enteroinvasive *E. coli*, *Yersinia* and *Listeria* are examples of bacteria that can invade human intestinal epithelial cells.[34–38] Enteropathogenic bacteria are particularly attractive models for the study of host–microbial interactions as they are subject to genetic manipulations that allow one to generate mutants that can be used to assess the relative importance of specific bacterial genes and gene products in the interaction with host epithelial cells. Moreover, different enteropathogenic bacteria have developed a range of strategies to infect host intestinal epithelial cells and also maintain distinct intracellular lifestyles during the course of epithelial cell invasion (e.g. either live free in the cytoplasm or live in vacuoles). This allows one to explore differences in early epithelial cell responses, as well as the coevolution of bacterial strategies and the host cellular response.[26]

One focus in our laboratory has been the role the intestinal epithelium can play in signaling or modulating host innate and acquired mucosal immunity. These studies have revealed different paradigms regarding how enteric microbes alter epithelial cell signaling and function following their interaction with host epithelial cells. We have used *in vitro* and *in vivo* model systems, mainly employing human intestinal epithelial cells. *In vitro* model systems include standard monolayer cultures of human intestinal epithelial cell lines, as well as the use of structurally and functionally polarized monolayers of human intestinal epithelium (i.e. the reductionist gut).[22,29,36,42,43] In regard to the latter, human intestinal epithelium is normally polarized into apical and basolateral domains, and information from polarized cultures of human intestinal epithelial cells (e.g. T84, Caco-2, HCA-7 cells) can yield important information regarding differences in apical and basolateral epithelial cell properties and functions that are relevant to host–microbial interactions.

An additional layer of complexity, and testing of the relevance of *in vitro* data, can be added through the use of *in vivo* model systems. One particularly useful *in vivo* model system has been the human fetal intestinal xenograft model. In this model, human fetal intestinal xenografts are transplanted subcutaneously on to the backs of severe combined immunodeficient (SCID) mice and allowed to mature for 10 weeks. The mature xenografts have an epithelium that is strictly of human origin.[44] This model is useful for exploring early changes in epithelial signaling in response to intraluminal infection of the xenografts or, alternatively, intestinal epithelial cell responses to signals delivered through epithelial cytokine receptors, including those whose expression is polarized to the basolateral epithelial cell membrane.[23,24,29,32,36,42,43] More complex *in vivo* systems take advantage of transgenic mice or chimeric 'knockout' mice in which specific genes have been overexpressed or deleted. In the future, other systems will be able to take advantage of mice in which genes have been conditionally altered in intestinal epithelial cells. It is important to note, however, that murine intestinal mucosal responses differ from those of humans to many of the pathogens known to cause mucosal inflammation and disease in the human intestine. It is also of note that advances in discovery-based research approaches are now available that enable one to more fully study the complete repertoire of epithelial cell responses to microbial infection using, for example, cDNA microarray analysis, as we initially showed for *Salmonella* infection of human colon epithelial cells.[37] Such approaches can reveal the activation of genes that might not otherwise be considered to be activated during infection, based on hypothesis-driven approaches.

Human intestinal epithelial cells have been shown to produce mediators essential for signaling the onset of acute mucosal inflammation in response to bacterial infection. For example, in response to infection with a number of enteroinvasive and some non-invasive bacterial pathogens that interact with the epithelial cell membrane, epithelial cells upregulate the production of potent chemoattractants for neutrophils (e.g. IL-8/CXCL8, GROα/CXCL1, GROβ/CXCL2, ENA78/CXCL5),[34,35,45] monocytes (e.g. MCP-1/CCL2),[45,46] and immature CCR6-expressing dendritic cells (MIP3α/CCL20).[36] Moreover, differences in the kinetics of upregulated chemokine expression and production by intestinal epithelial cells, and differences in the functional properties of chemokines that have similar targets, may result in spatial and temporal chemokine gradients for the chemoattraction of target inflammatory cells within the intestinal mucosa.[45]

Signaling within intestinal epithelial cells that is initiated by a broad array of different bacterial pathogens with different strategies for epithelial cell entry and different intracellular lifestyles converges to activate the transcription factor NF-κB and its target genes,[38] including the above-mentioned chemokine genes.[36,38] This has led to the concept that NF-κB is a central regulator of epithelial cell signaling pathways essential for initiating host innate immune responses to microbial pathogens.[38] Activation of the I-κ kinase (IKK) complex, and notably the IKKβ subunit, is an essential step in the activation of NF-κB by a number of enteric pathogens and by proinflammatory mediators. Moreover, some pathogens (e.g. *Yersinia*), through their type III secretory proteins, have developed strategies to prevent the activation of NF-κB and other signal transduction pathways, and consequently to modulate the resultant host inflammatory response.[47,48]

Recent studies have also begun to elucidate the role the epithelium can play in providing signals important for the development of mucosal adaptive immunity. In this regard, the small intestinal epithelium constitutively produces TECK/CCL25, whose cognate receptor CCR9 is expressed on $\alpha_4\beta_7$ expressing T cells that preferentially localize to the small intestinal mucosa.[49,50] In contrast, colon epithelial cells do not produce

TECK/CCL25, but do produce MEC/CCL28, whose cognate ligand is CCR10.[51,52] Thus, subpopulations of CCR10-expressing cells preferentially localize to sites of MEC production in the gut (e.g. colon, salivary glands). Such chemokines appear to be important for the selective migration of lymphocyte subsets to the small intestine and colon, respectively.

Under inflammatory conditions, human intestinal epithelial cells can produce IFN-γ-inducible chemokines (e.g. Mig/CCL9, IP-10/CCL10, I-TAC/CCL11)[42,53] that chemoattract CXCR3-expressing T cells that have a memory phenotype, and themselves produce the Th1-type cytokine IFN-γ, and MDC/CCL22,[43] a chemoattractant for CCR4-expressing cells. Whereas the IFN-γ inducible chemokines CCL9, CCL10 and CCL11 are not substantially upregulated in intestinal epithelial cells in response to bacterial infection alone, their upregulation by IFN-γ stimulation is synergistically increased by concurrent bacterial infection.[42] Conversely, upregulated epithelial cell expression of MDC/CCL22 by intestinal epithelial cells, which ensues in response to bacterial infection, is synergistically increased by IFN-γ.[43] Thus, microbial infection that takes place in the milieu of other mucosal inflammatory processes appears to markedly potentiate the ability of the epithelial cells to

produce chemokines important for signaling cells that play a role in host adaptive immune responses. Intestinal epithelial cells notably do not express several cytokines key in regulating adaptive immune responses (e.g. IL-2, IL-4, IFN-γ, IL-12p40)[34,35] (Figure 12.3).

Conclusion

In summary, emerging evidence indicates that the surface epithelium lining the human small intestine and colon has developed highly sophisticated mechanisms to interact with enteric microbes (Figure 12.4). These mechanisms play key roles in:

- intraluminal host defense;
- signaling the onset of mucosal innate immunity;
- setting the stage for host adaptive immune responses by ensuring that the appropriate cell populations are brought into the intestinal mucosa;
- linking the onset of mucosal innate and adaptive immune responses. For the most part, intestinal epithelial cell responses appear to have coevolved with microbial strategies, and many intestinal epithelial cell responses can be regarded to be of benefit both to the host and to the microbe during its interaction with the host.

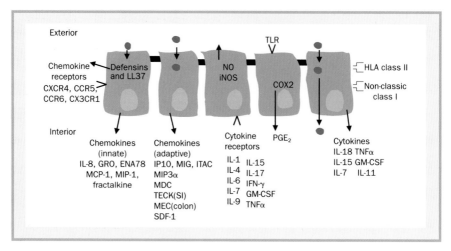

Figure 12.3
Epithelial cells are important for innate and adaptive immunity.

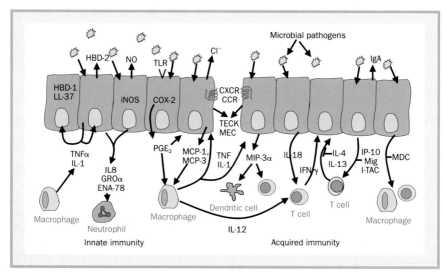

Figure 12.4
Role of the intestinal epithelium in defending against enteric infections.

References

1. Rescigno M, Urbano M, Valzasina B, *et al*. Dendritic cells express tight junction proteins and penetrate gut epithelial monolayers to sample bacteria. *Nature Immunol* 2001; 2: 361–367.

2. Neutra MR, Mantis NJ, Frey A, Giannasca PJ. The composition and function of M cell apical membranes: implications for microbial pathogenesis. *Semin Immunol* 1999; 11: 171–181.

3. Sansonetti PJ. Rupture, invasion and inflammatory destruction of the intestinal barrier by Shigella, making sense of prokaryote-eukaryote cross-talks. *FEMS Microbiol Rev* 2001; 25:3–14.

4. Kim JM, Eckmann L, Savidge TC, Lowe DC, Witthoft T, Kagnoff MF. Apoptosis of human intestinal epithelial cells after bacterial invasion. *J Clin Invest* 1998; 102:1815–1823.

5. McCole DF, Eckmann L, Laurent F, Kagnoff MF. Intestinal epithelial cell apoptosis following *Cryptosporidium parvum* infection. *Infect Immun* 2000; 68:1710–1713.

6. Fan T, Lu H, Hu H, *et al*. Inhibition of apoptosis in chlamydia-infected cells: blockade of mitochondrial cytochrome c release and caspase activation. *J Exp Med* 1998; 187:487–496.

7. Varilek GW, Neil GA, Bishop WP. Caco-2 cells express type I interleukin-1 receptors: ligand binding enhances proliferation. *Am J Physiol* 1994; 267:G1101–1107.

8. Colgan SP, Resnick MB, Parkos CA, *et al*. IL-4 directly modulates function of a model human intestinal epithelium. *J Immunol* 1994; 153:2122–2129.

9. Reinecker HC, Podolsky DK. Human intestinal epithelial cells express functional cytokine receptors sharing the common γc chain of the interleukin 2 receptor. *Proc Natl Acad Sci USA* 1995; 92:8353–8357.

10. Reinecker HC, MacDermott RP, Mirau S, Dignass A, Podolsky DK. Intestinal epithelial cells both express and respond to interleukin 15. *Gastroenterology* 1996; 111:1706–1713.

11. Yamada K, Shimaoka M, Nagayama K, Hiroi T, Kiyono H, Honda T. Bacterial invasion induces interleukin-7 receptor expression in colonic epithelial cell line, T84. *Eur J Immunol* 1997; 27:3456–3460.

12. Panja A, Goldberg S, Eckmann L, Krishen P, Mayer L. The regulation and functional consequence of proinflammatory cytokine binding on human intestinal epithelial cells. *J Immunol* 1998; 161:3675–3684.

13. Fish SM, Proujansky R, Reenstra WW. Synergistic effects of interferon gamma and tumour necrosis factor-α on T84 cell function. *Gut* 1999; 45:191–198.

14. Awane M, Andres PG, Li DJ, Reinecker HC. NF-κB-inducing kinase is a common mediator of IL-17-, TNF-α, and IL-1β-induced chemokine promoter activation in intestinal epithelial cells. *J Immunol* 1999; 162:5337–5344.

15. Denning TL, Campbell NA, Song F, *et al*. Expression of IL-10 receptors on epithelial cells from the murine small and large intestine. *Int Immunol* 2000; 12:133–139.

16. Dwinell MB, Eckmann L, Leopard JD, Varki NM, Kagnoff MF. Chemokine receptor expression by human intestinal epithelial cells. *Gastroenterology* 1999; 117:359–367.

17. Delezay O, Koch N, Yahi N, *et al*. Co-expression of CXCR4/fusin and galactosylceramide in the human intestinal epithelial cell line HT-29. *AIDS* 1997; 11: 1311–1318.

18. Jordan NJ, Kolios G, Abbot SE, *et al.* Expression of functional CXCR4 chemokine receptors on human colonic epithelial cells. *J Clin Invest* 1999; 104:1061–1069.

19. Cario E, Rosenberg IM, Brandwein SL, Beck PL, Reinecker HC, Podolsky DK. Lipopolysaccharide activates distinct signaling pathways in intestinal epithelial cell lines expressing Toll-like receptors. *J Immunol* 2000; 64:966–972.

20. Steinle A, Groh V, Spies T. Diversification, expression, and gamma delta T cell recognition of evolutionarily distant members of the MIC family of major histocompatibility complex class I-related molecules. *Proc Natl Acad Sci USA* 1998; 95:12510–12515.

21. Colgan SP, Hershberg RM, Furuta GT, Blumberg RS. Ligation of intestinal epithelial CD1d induces bioactive IL-10: critical role of the cytoplasmic tail in autocrine signaling. *Proc Natl Acad Sci USA* 1999; 96: 13938–13943.

22. Witthoft T, Eckmann L, Kim JM, Kagnoff MF. Enteroinvasive bacteria directly activate expression of iNOS and NO production in human colon epithelial cells. *Am J Physiol* 1998; 275:G564–G671.

23. Eckmann L, Stenson WF, Savidge TC, *et al.* Role of intestinal epithelial cells in the host secretory response to infection by invasive bacteria. Bacterial entry induces epithelial prostaglandin H synthase-2 expression and prostaglandin E_2 and $F_{2\alpha}$ production. *J Clin Invest* 1997; 100:296–309.

24. O'Neil DA, Porter EM, Elewaut D, *et al.* Expression and regulation of the human β-defensins hBD-1 and hBD-2 in intestinal epithelium. *J Immunol* 1999; 163:6718–6724.

25. O'Neil DA, Cole SP, Martin-Porter E, *et al.* Regulation of human β-defensins by gastric epithelial cells in response to infection with Helicobacter pylori or stimulation with interleukin-1. *Infect Immun* 2000; 68: 5412–5415.

26. Kagnoff MF, Eckmann L. Epithelial cells as sensors for microbial infection. *J Clin Invest* 1997; 100:6–10.

27. Eckmann L, Laurent F, Langford TD, *et al.* Nitric oxide production by human intestinal epithelial cells and competition for arginine as potential determinants of host defense against the lumen-dwelling pathogen *Giardia lamblia.* *J Immunol* 2000; 164:1478–1487.

28. Rasmussen SJ, Eckmann L, Quayle AJ, *et al.* Secretion of proinflammatory cytokines by epithelial cells in response to *Chlamydia* infection suggests a central role for epithelial cells in chlamydial pathogenesis. *J Clin Invest* 1997; 99:77–87.

29. Laurent F, Eckmann L, Savidge TC, *et al.* *Cryptosporidium parvum* infection of human intestinal epithelial cells induces the polarized secretion of C-X-C chemokines. *Infect Immun* 1997; 65:5067–5073.

30. Laurent F, Kagnoff MF, Savidge TC, Naciri M, Eckmann L. Human intestinal epithelial cells respond to *Cryptosporidium parvum* infection with increased prostaglandin H synthase 2 expression and prostaglandin E_2 and $F_{2\alpha}$ production. *Infect Immun* 1998; 66: 1787–1790.

31. Laurent F, McCole D, Eckmann L, Kagnoff MF. Pathogenesis of *Cryptosporidium parvum* infection. *Microbes Infect* 1999; 1:141–148.

32. Huang GT, Eckmann L, Savidge TC, Kagnoff MF. Infection of human intestinal epithelial cells with invasive bacteria upregulates apical intercellular adhesion

molecule-1 (ICAM)-1) expression and neutrophil adhesion. *J Clin Invest* 1996; 98: 572–583.

33. Eckmann L, Reed SL, Smith JR, Kagnoff MF. Entamoeba histolytica trophozoites induce an inflammatory cytokine response by cultured human cells through the paracrine action of cytolytically released interleukin-1α. *J Clin Invest* 1995; 96:1269–1279.

34. Jung HC, Eckmann L, Yang SK, *et al.* A distinct array of proinflammatory cytokines is expressed in human colon epithelial cells in response to bacterial invasion. *J Clin Invest* 1995; 95:55–65.

35. Eckmann L, Kagnoff MF, Fierer J. Epithelial cells secrete the chemokine interleukin-8 in response to bacterial entry. *Infect Immun* 1993; 61:4569–4574.

36. Izadpanah A, Dwinell MB, Eckmann L, Varki NM, Kagnoff MF. Regulated MIP-3α/CCL20 production by human intestinal epithelium: mechanism for modulating mucosal immunity. *Am J Physiol Gastrointest Liver Physiol.* 2001; 280:G710–9.

37. Eckmann L, Smith JR, Housley MP, Dwinell MB, Kagnoff MF. Analysis by high density cDNA arrays of altered gene expression in human intestinal epithelial cells in response to infection with the invasive enteric bacteria *Salmonella. J Biol Chem* 2000; 275: 14084–14094.

38. Elewaut D, DiDonato JA, Kim JM, Truong F, Eckmann L, Kagnoff MF. NF-κB is a central regulator of the intestinal epithelial cell innate immune response induced by infection with enteroinvasive bacteria. *J Immunol* 1999; 163:1457–1466.

39. Eckmann L, Rudolf MT, Ptasznik A, *et al.* D-myo-Inositol 1,4,5,6-tetrakisphosphate produced in human intestinal epithelial cells in response to *Salmonella* invasion inhibits phosphoinositide 3-kinase signaling pathways. *Proc Natl Acad Sci USA* 1997; 94: 14456–14460.

40. Savkovic SD, Koutsouris A, Hecht G. Activation of NF-κB in intestinal epithelial cells by enteropathogenic *Escherichia coli. Am J Physiol* 1997; 273:C1160–1167.

41. Hecht G, Marrero JA, Danilkovich A, *et al. Pathogenic Escherichia* coli increase Cl- secretion from intestinal epithelia by upregulating galanin-1 receptor expression. *J Clin Invest* 1999; 104:253–262.

42. Dwinell MB, Lugering N, Eckmann L, Kagnoff MF. Regulated production of interferon-inducible T-cell chemoattractants by human intestinal epithelial cells. *Gastroenterology* 2001; 120:49–59.

43. Berin MC, Dwinell MB, Eckmann L, Kagnoff, MF. Production of MDC/CCL22 by human intestinal epithelial cells. *Am J Physiol Gastrointest Liver Physiol* 2001; 280: G1217.

44. Shmakov AN, Morey AL, Ferguson DJ, Fleming KA, O'Brien JA, Savidge TC. Conventional patterns of human intestinal proliferation in a severe-combined immunodeficient xenograft model. *Differentiation* 1995; 59:321–330.

45. Yang SK, Eckmann L, Panja A, Kagnoff MF. Differential and regulated expression of C-X-C, C-C, and C-chemokines by human colon epithelial cells. *Gastroenterology* 1997; 113: 1214–1223.

46. Reinecker HC, Loh EY, Ringler DJ, Mehta A, Rombeau JL, MacDermott RP. Monocyte-chemoattractant protein 1 gene expression in intestinal epithelial cells and inflammatory

bowel disease mucosa. *Gastroenterology* 1995; 108:40–50.

47. Schesser K, Spiik AK, Dukuzumuremyi JM, Neurath MF, Pettersson S, Wolf-Watz H. The yopJ locus is required for *Yersinia*-mediated inhibition of NF-κB activation and cytokine expression: YopJ contains a eukaryotic SH2-like domain that is essential for its repressive activity. *Mol Microbiol* 1998; 28:1067–1079.

48. Meijer LK, Schesser K, Wolf-Watz H, Sassone-Corsi P, Pettersson S. The bacterial protein YopJ abrogates multiple signal transduction pathways that converge on the transcription factor CREB. *Cell Microbiol* 2000; 2:231–238.

49. Wurbel MA, Philippe JM, Nguyen C, *et al.* The chemokine TECK is expressed by thymic and intestinal epithelial cells and attracts double- and single-positive thymocytes expressing the TECK receptor CCR9. *Eur J Immunol* 2000; 30:262–271.

50. Kunkel EJ, Campbell JJ, Haraldsen G, *et al.* Lymphocyte CC chemokine receptor 9 and epithelial thymus-expressed chemokine (TECK) expression distinguish the small intestinal immune compartment: epithelial expression of tissue-specific chemokines as an organizing principle in regional immunity. *J Exp Med* 2000; 192:761–768.

51. Wang W, Soto H, Oldham ER, *et al.* Identification of a novel chemokine (CCL28), which binds CCR10 (GPR2). *J Biol Chem* 2000; 275:22313–22323.

52. Pan J, Kunkel EJ, Gosslar U, *et al.* A novel chemokine ligand for CCR10 and CCR3 expressed by epithelial cells in mucosal tissues. *J Immunol* 2000; 165:2943–2949.

53. Shibahara T, Wilcox JN, Couse T, Madara JL. Characterization of epithelial chemoattractants for human intestinal intraepithelial lymphocytes. *Gastroenterology* 2001; 120:60–70.

Summary and observations

R Balfour Sartor

Part 4 has highlighted the interaction of luminal bacteria with the host's epithelial cell and mucosal immune system response. The host's innate and acquired immune response to invading and commensal enteric bacteria determines effective clearance of pathogenic microbial species versus chronic infection, and homeostatic immunologic tolerance versus chronic inflammation.

In addition, Part 4 elegantly reviews mechanisms of intestinal epithelial cell responses to invading bacteria and parasites using both *in vitro* cultured colonic epithelial cell lines and explants of fetal intestines in immunodeficient mice. Bacterial and parasitic invasion stimulates a programmed innate immune response in the epithelial cell with a characteristic profile of chemokines, MHC Class II molecules, and adhesion molecules that recruit neutrophils, monocyte/macrophages and T lymphocytes to the invaded mucosal surface. These inflammatory molecules are transcriptionally regulated by NFκB. In this manner, intestinal epithelial cells function as sentinels and, when activated, initiate a sequence of events culminating in the recruitment of effector cells to the invaded mucosal surface which clear the invading organism.

The profound influence of commensal luminal bacteria on induction of protective mucosal immune responses in normal hosts is also described, in addition to the stimulation of cell-mediated chronic inflammation in genetically susceptible hosts with defective mucosal barrier function or disordered immunoregulation. Some provocative experimental data suggest that the enteric Gram-negative bacteria preferentially induce immunologic tolerance at the mucosal surface, which is mediated by

IL-10 and TGFß. In contrast, susceptible hosts, including genetically engineered knockout and transgenic rodents, develop chronic mucosal inflammation when colonized with normal bacteria, and remain free of disease when raised in a sterile environment. Of considerable interest, some commensal bacteria preferentially induce inflammation and Th1 immune responses, and host genetic background appears to determine selectivity of the bacterial stimulus.

The evolving concept of dysbiosis, or altered composition of commensal bacteria, in hosts with chronic inflammation is discussed, as is the use of novel molecular methods, which have dramatically expanded our ability to dissect the complex microecology of the distal intestine. Finally, Part 4 examines the ability of probiotic bacterial species to stimulate protective mucosal immune responses and to prevent experimental and clinical intestinal inflammation.

These concepts help explain the mechanisms by which the host responds to enteric microbial colonization, leading to either protective or pathologic consequences. These insights can be used for precise therapeutic interventions that amplify protective responses or selectively block detrimental processes.

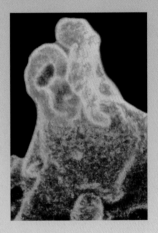

PART 5
Modification of the intestinal flora

Modification of gut microflora: a novel treatment target in childhood disease

Erika Isolauri and Seppo Salminen

13

Introduction

The mucosa of the gastrointestinal tract functions as a barrier, excluding numerous antigens derived from microorganisms and food. In intestinal inflammation, the integrity of the barrier is disrupted and antigens are able to traverse the mucosal barrier. This may evoke aberrant immune responses and the release of proinflammatory cytokines, with further impairment of the barrier function.

The recent demonstration that the gut microflora is an important constituent of the intestine's mucosal barrier has introduced new therapeutic strategies for combating enteric infections in children, and possibly other intestinal inflammatory conditions. The potential modification of the intestinal flora to increase the predominance of specific non-pathogenic bacteria and modify the intestinal milieu thus seems a reasonable topic for future research. The experimental approaches so far include local delivery of specific bacteria engineered to produce anti-inflammatory cytokines and probiotic therapy. So far, the best-documented clinical application is the treatment of acute diarrhoea by specific probiotic bacteria. In humans, documented effects have also been reported for alleviation of intestinal inflammation, normalisation of gut mucosal dysfunction, and downregulation of hypersensitivity reactions. Recent data indicate that differences in immunomodulatory effects exist between candidate probiotic bacteria. Distinct regulatory effects have been detected in healthy subjects and patients with inflammatory diseases. These results suggest that specific immunomodulatory properties of probiotic bacteria should be characterised during the development of clinical applications for extended target populations. As probiotics offer a tool for modification of gut barrier and microflora, the microbes used have to be obtained from acceptable sources with a proven safety record and efficacy to guarantee their application for food and therapeutic use.

Normal gut microflora in development

At birth the gastrointestinal tract of the newborn is sterile. The maternal intestinal flora is the first source of colonising bacteria. Colonisation is also determined by contact with the surroundings. At this stage, the dominating strains are facultative anaerobes, such as the enterobacteria, coliforms and lactobacilli.[1] Thereafter, differences exist in the composition of species, due mainly to the type of diet. Breastfeeding encourages the

growth of bifidobacteria, while formula-fed infants have a more complex microflora, with bifidobacteria, enterobacteria, lactobacilli, bacteroides, clostridia and streptococci. After weaning, the composition of the microflora resembles that of the adult flora. Although bacteria are distributed throughout the intestine, the major concentration of microbes and metabolic activity can be found in the large intestine. From culture-based data it is thought that at least 500 different microbial species exist, although on a quantitative basis, 10–20 genera probably predominate: *Bacteroides, Lactobacillus, Clostridium, Fusobacterium, Bifidobacterium, Eubacterium, Peptococcus, Peptostreptococcus, Escherichia* and *Veillonella.*[2]

The indigenous bacteria have sometimes been classified as either potentially pathogenic or as health-promoting in nature.[2] The strains with beneficial properties include bifidobacteria and lactobacilli. In infectious and inflammatory conditions the balance of the gut microecology is altered in such a way that the number of potentially pathogenic bacteria increases.[2,3] The commonest probiotics are bifidobacteria and lactobacilli, which exert powerful antipathogenic capabilities and are mainly responsible for colonisation resistance in the gut. Moreover, the same genera have been attributed with other beneficial aspects, such as stimulation of the immune response, thereby promoting non-specific host resistance to microbial pathogens.

Gut microflora and intestinal inflammation

Altered gut microecology is reported in many inflammatory diseases. Rotavirus diarrhoea is associated with an increased concentration of faecal urease, an inflammatory mediator, which predisposes the gut mucosa to ammonia-induced destruction and to the overgrowth of urease-producing bacteria.[4] Duchmann *et al.*[5] have demonstrated that healthy individuals are tolerant to their own microflora, and that such tolerance is abrogated in patients with inflammatory bowel disease. Altered gut microflora is reported in patients with rheumatoid arthritis[6] and allergic disease,[7,8] implying that the gut normal microflora constitutes an ecosystem responding to inflammation in the gut and elsewhere in the human body.

Normalisation of the properties of the indigenous microflora by specific strains of the healthy gut microflora forms the basis of probiotic therapy. Oral introduction of probiotics may halt the vicious circle by normalising the increased intestinal permeability and altered gut microecology, improving the intestine's immunological barrier functions and alleviating the intestinal inflammatory response. The targets for probiotic therapy are thus clinical conditions with impaired mucosal barrier function, particularly infectious and inflammatory disease.[9]

Modification of gut microflora and treatment of disease

In intestinal infectious, inflammatory and allergic conditions the experimental therapeutic approaches include the local delivery of specific bacteria engineered to produce anti-inflammatory cytokines and probiotic therapy. Dietary administration of *Lactococcus lactis*, genetically engineered to produce the anti-inflammatory interleukin-10 (IL-10), was shown to be effective in a mouse model of inflammatory bowel disease.[10]

The future of the application of gut microflora modulation in human nutrition and in the science of functional foods clearly lies in clinical demonstrations. Thus, the potential health effects of normal gut microflora have to be demonstrated by well-controlled clinical and nutritional studies in human subjects. In human disease, data on the therapeutic potential of probiotics have been accumulating.[2]

The principal effect of probiotics is characterised by stabilisation of the gut microflora.[2] Clinical benefit is demonstrated in conditions in which the gut microecology is disturbed by changes in the environment (travellers' diarrhoea) or by oral antimicrobial therapy (antibiotic-associated diarrhoea). The most extensively studied gastrointestinal condition treated by probiotics is acute infantile diarrhoea. In patients hospitalised for acute rotavirus diarrhoea, *Lactobacillus* strain

GG (ATCC 53103), in the form of either fermented milk or a freeze-dried powder, significantly reduced the duration of diarrhoea compared to the placebo group given pasteurised yogurt.[11] The result has been confirmed in studies carried out in a similar population,[12] as well as in different populations.[13] The multicentre study of the European Society for Paediatric Gastroenterology, Hepatology and Nutrition working group tested the clinical effect of probiotics on acute diarrhoea caused by rotavirus or other pathogens.[14] In rotavirus diarrhoea a significant shortening in the duration of illness was observed, while in non-specific or bacterial diarrhoea no clear effect was found. The demonstration that this probiotic was safe and caused a significant reduction in the duration of diarrhoea and hospitalisation as well as prevention of the evolution of rotavirus diarrhoea towards a protracted course provides evidence-based documentation for the treatment of rotavirus diarrhoea in infants by probiotics.

The beneficial clinical effect of probiotic therapy has been explained by stabilisation of the indigenous microflora,[4] reduction in the duration of rotavirus shedding[15] and reduction in increased gut permeability caused by rotavirus infection,[16] together with a significant increase in immunoglobulin A (IgA)-secreting cells to rotavirus.[17,18]

There is an increasing appreciation of the role of cytokines in regulating the inflam-matory responses at the local and systemic level. Ingestion of probiotic bacteria has the potential to stabilise the immunological barrier in the gut mucosa by reducing the generation of local proinflammatory cytokines.[9] Alteration of the properties of the indigenous microflora by probiotic therapy has been shown to reverse some immunological disturbances characteristic of Crohn's disease[19] and food allergy.[20] Recently, a significant improvement in the clinical course of atopic dermatitis (eczema) in infants given a probiotic-supplemented elimination diet was detected and, in parallel, markers of intestinal-[20] and systemic-[21] allergic inflammation decreased significantly. Similar results have been obtained in milk-hypersensitive adults.[22] In these, a milk challenge in conjunction with a probiotic strain prevented the immunoinflammatory response characteristic of the challenge without probiotics.

Modification of gut microflora in reducing the risk of human disease

The role of the diet in health and wellbeing has changed as the science of nutrition has evolved. The principal role is clearly the provision of energy to meet the requirements of metabolism and growth. However, research interest is directed towards the improvement of specific physiological effects of the diet beyond its nutritional impact. In particular, the potential role of functional foods to reduce the risk of diseases has been assessed.[2] A food can be regarded as 'functional' if it is shown to affect beneficially one or more target functions in the body, beyond adequate nutritional effects, in a way which is relevant to either the state of wellbeing and health and/or to the reduction of the risk of disease.[2]

The best-documented application of probiotics in the reduction of the risk of human disease is the prevention of acute infantile diarrhoea. Saavedra *et al.*[23] conducted a double-blind placebo-controlled trial in hospitalised infants who were randomised to receive a standard infant formula or the same formula supplemented with *Bifidobacterium bifidum* (later renamed *Bifidobacterium lactis*) and *Streptococcus thermophilus*. Over a 17-month follow-up, 31% of the patients given the standard infant formula, but only 7% of those receiving the probiotic-supplemented formula developed diarrhoea, and the prevalence of rotavirus shedding was significantly lower in those receiving probiotic-supplemented formula. More recently, Szajewska *et al.*[24] evaluated the efficacy of orally administered *Lactobacillus* GG in the prevention of nosocomial diarrhoea in young children. Eighty-one children aged 1–36 months who were hospitalised for reasons other than diarrhoea were enrolled in a randomised double-blind trial to receive

probiotics or placebo for the duration of their hospital stay. *Lactobacillus* GG reduced the risk of nosocomial diarrhoea compared with placebo (6.7% vs 33.3%; relative risk: 0.2; [95% CI: 0.06–0.6]). The prevalence of rotavirus infection was similar in probiotic and placebo groups. However, the use of probiotics rather than placebo significantly reduced the risk of rotavirus gastroenteritis, suggesting that probiotics reduce the risk of nosocomial diarrhoea in infants, particularly nosocomial rotavirus gastroenteritis.

The role of the intestinal microflora in oral tolerance induction – the unresponsiveness to non-pathogenic antigens encountered at the mucosal surface – to the IgE response has been recently investigated in germ-free mice.[25] In contrast to control mice, germ-free animals maintained their tendency to systemic immune response, such as the production of IgE antibodies, upon oral administration of ovalbumin. Abrogation of oral tolerance was due to the lack of intestinal flora. The aberrant IgE response in germ-free mice could be corrected by reconstitution of the microflora at the neonatal stage, but not later. These results suggest that by altering the development of gut-associated lymphoid tissue at an early age, the gut microflora directs the regulation of systemic and local immune responsiveness. Parallel results have been obtained in humans. Recent studies following the microfloral development in vaginally born infants and in infants born by caesarean section showed major differences in culturable microflora.[26] Colonisation was associated with the maturation of humoral immune mechanisms, particularly of circulating IgA- and IgM-secreting cells.[27]

Modification of the gut microflora in allergic disease

The regulatory role of probiotics in human allergic disease was first emphasised in a demonstration of a suppressive effect on lymphocyte proliferation and interleukin-4 generation *in vitro*.[28,29] Subsequently, the immunoinflammatory responses to dietary antigens in allergic individuals were shown to be alleviated by probiotics, this being partly attributable to enhanced production of anti-inflammatory cytokines, e.g. interleukin-10[30] and transforming growth factor-β,[21] and partly to control of allergic inflammation in the gut.[20]

The role of the exposure to commensal microflora as a key modulator of the human immune system against atopy and atopic diseases was recently evaluated.[31] Intestinal microflora from 76 infants at high risk of atopic diseases were analysed at 3 weeks and 3 months of age by conventional bacterial cultivation and two culture-independent methods, gas–liquid chromatography of bacterial cellular fatty acids and quantitative fluorescence *in situ* hybridisation of bacterial cells. Atopy was diagnosed if the infants

evinced at least one positive skin prick reaction at 12 months, and those with negative skin prick tests were defined as non-atopic. Atopic sensitisation was observed in 22/76 (29%) children. At 3 weeks the bacterial cellular fatty acid profile in faecal samples differed significantly between infants developing and those not developing atopy ($P = 0.005$). By fluorescence *in situ* hybridisation, atopics had more clostridia and fewer bifidobacteria in their stools than non-atopics, resulting in a reduced ratio of bifidobacteria to clostridia ($P = 0.03$). Differences in the neonatal gut microflora were thus shown to precede the development of atopy, suggesting a crucial role for the balance of indigenous intestinal bacteria in the maturation of human immunity to a non-atopic mode. Indeed, as documented in the first clinical report of the allergy prevention project of the authors, probiotics administered pre- and postnatally for 6 months to children at high risk of atopic diseases, succeeded in reducing the prevalence of atopic eczema to half, compared with that in infants receiving placebo.[32]

Safety aspects – the focus of future research

Probiotics form a relatively new treatment modality for gastrointestinal disorders. The ingestion of large numbers of viable bacteria requires an assurance of safety. Probiotics have been selected from members of the normal healthy intestinal microflora, but new probiotic microbes have recently been introduced. Currently used probiotics have been deemed safe for use in fermented foods, but generally the safety assessment of microbial food supplements is not well developed.[33]

Studies have suggested the gut as an origin of disease caused by bacteria normally residing in the intestinal lumen but occasionally translocating across the intestinal epithelium.[34] Translocation may be enhanced by gut barrier and microflora dysfunction caused by inflammation. Effective probiotics may have properties that counteract the epithelial damage. The concept of translocation sets specific safety requirements for microbes used for oral bacteriotherapy.[35] Among these are the origin, species characteristics and stability of strain properties. An acceptable origin has been defined by focusing on microbes that are members of the normal healthy human intestinal microflora. Bifidobacteria and lactic acid bacteria are generally regarded as normal constituents of the intestinal flora. They have rarely caused disease through translocation and their safety record through use in fermented milk, vegetables and cereals is excellent. Their natural presence in all human mucosal surfaces also attests to their safety. For future new probiotics, it is important to assess their specific properties relating to

translocation potential. These include resistance to complement-mediated killing and phagocytosis, haemagglutination, haemolysis and platelet aggregation.[36] Their influence and long-term effects on the resident gut microflora and its metabolic activity should be characterised.

Genetically modified microorganisms are currently not used or planned for use in foods. The rapid development in this area may change their application targets. Reports on the effects of *Lactococcus lactis* engineered to locally produce interleukin-10 in mouse intestinal mucosa points to a strong potential for future therapeutic applications.[10] The most important safety factor is the content of antibiotic resistance markers in the genetic constituents of modified organisms. Selection procedures have been developed to ensure such safety prerequisite specifically for lactococci.[36] For the genetically modified organisms, the European novel food legislation sets the criteria that must be tested prior to the introduction to foods or therapeutic products. Studies should emphasise the modified property and its potential health effects, in both the short and long term. These safety criteria, together with the demonstration of efficacy, form the future direction for therapeutic modification of gut microflora in general, and the use of selected natural or engineered probiotics in particular.

Conclusions

Probiotic therapy is based on the concept of a healthy microflora. Probiotics can help stabilise the gut microbial environment and the intestine's permeability barrier, and enhance systemic and mucosal IgA responses, thereby promoting the immunological barrier of gut mucosa. The probiotic approach – therapeutic consumption of cultures of beneficial microorganisms of the healthy human microflora – holds great promise for the treatment of clinical conditions associated with impaired gut mucosal barrier functions and sustained inflammatory responses. The future focus of nutrition emphasises health and wellbeing. Probiotic modulation of intestinal microflora promotes this and aims to reduce the risk of gut-associated diseases.

References

1. Benno Y, Mitsuoka T. Development of intestinal microflora in humans and animals. *Bifidobacteria Microfi* 1986; 5:13–25.

2. Salminen S, Bouley C, Boutron-Ruault MC, *et al.* Gastrointestinal physiology and function – targets for functional food development. *Br J Nutr* 1998; 80(Suppl):147–171.

3. Isolauri E. Probiotics and gut inflammation. *Curr Opin Gastroenterol* 1999; 15:534–537.

4. Isolauri E, Kaila M, Mykkänen H, *et al.* Oral bacteriotherapy for viral gastroenteritis. *Dig Dis Sci* 1994; 39:2595–2600.

5. Duchmann R, Kaiser I, Hermann E, *et al.* Tolerance exists towards resident intestinal flora but is broken in active inflammatory bowel disease (IBD). *Clin Exp Immunol* 1995; 102:448–455.

6. Malin M, Verronen P, Mykkänen H, *et al.* Increased bacterial urease activity in faeces in juvenile chronic arthritis: evidence of altered intestinal microflora? *Br J Rheumatol* 1996; 35:689–694.

7. Apostolou E, Pelto L, Kirjavainen PV, *et al.* Differences in the gut bacterial flora of healthy and milk-hypersensitive adults, as measured by fluorescence in situ hybridisation. *FEMS Immunol Med Microbiol* 2001; 31:35–39.

8. Björkstén B, Naaber P, Sepp E, *et al.* The intestinal microflora in allergic Estonian and Swedish 2-year-old children. *Clin Exp Allergy* 1999; 29:342–346.

9. Isolauri E, Sütas Y, Kankaanpää P, *et al.* Probiotics: effects on immunity. *Am J Clin Nutr* 2001; 73:S444–S450.

10. Steidler L, Hans W, Schotte L, *et al.* Treatment of murine colitis by *Lactococcus lactis* secreting interleukin-10. *Science* 2000; 289:1352–1355.

11. Isolauri E, Juntunen M, Rautanen T, *et al.* A human *Lactobacillus* strain (*Lactobacillus* GG) promotes recovery from acute diarrhoea in children. *Pediatrics* 1991; 88:90–97.

12. Majamaa H, Isolauri E, Saxelin M, *et al.* Lactic acid bacteria in the treatment of acute rotavirus gastroenteritis. *J Pediatr Gastroenterol Nutr* 1995; 20:333–339.

13. Pant AR, Graham SM, Allen SJ, *et al.* *Lactobacillus* GG and acute diarrhoea in young children in the tropics. *J Trop Pediatr* 1996; 42:162–165.

14. Guandalini S, Pensabene L, Zikri MA, *et al.* *Lactobacillus* GG administered in oral rehydration solution to children with acute

diarrhoea: a multicenter European trial. *J Pediatr Gastroenterol Nutr* 2000; 30:54–60.

15. Canani RB, Albano F, Spagnuolo MI, *et al.* Effect of oral administration of *Lactobacillus* GG on the duration of diarrhoea and on rotavirus excretion in ambulatory children. *J Pediatr Gastroenterol Nutr* 1997; 24:469.

16. Isolauri E, Kaila M, Arvola T, *et al.* Diet during rotavirus enteritis affects jejunal permeability to macromolecules in suckling rats. *Pediatr Res* 1993; 33:548–553.

17. Kaila M, Isolauri E, Soppi E, *et al.* Enhancement of the circulating antibody secreting cell response in human diarrhoea by a human lactobacillus strain. *Pediatr Res* 1992; 32:141–144.

18. Isolauri E, Majamaa H, Arvola T, *et al. Lactobacillus casei* strain GG reverses increased intestinal permeability induced by cow milk in suckling rats. *Gastroenterology* 1993; 105:1643–1650.

19. Malin M, Suomalainen H, Saxelin M, *et al.* Promotion of IgA immune response in patients with Crohn's disease by oral bacteriotherapy with *Lactobacillus* GG. *Ann Nutr Metab* 1996; 40:137–145.

20. Majamaa H, Isolauri E. Probiotics: a novel approach in the management of food allergy. *J Allergy Clin Immunol* 1997; 99:179–186.

21. Isolauri E, Arvola T, Sütas Y, *et al.* Probiotics in the management of atopic eczema. *Clin Exp Allergy* 2000; 30:1605–1610.

22. Pelto L, Isolauri E, Lilius EM, *et al.* Probiotic bacteria downregulate the milk-induced inflammatory response in milk-hypersensitive subjects but have an immunostimulatory effect in healthy subjects. *Clin Exp Allergy* 1998; 28:1474–1479.

23. Saavedra JM, Bauman NA, Oung I, *et al.*

Feeding of *Bifidobacterium bifidum* and *Streptococcus thermophilus* to infants in hospital for prevention of diarrhoea and shedding of rotavirus. *Lancet* 1994; 344: 1046–1409.

24. Szajewska H, Kotowska M, Mrukowicz JZ, *et al.* Efficacy of *Lactobacillus* GG in prevention of nosocomial diarrhoea in infants. *J Pediatr* 2001; 138:361–365.

25. Sudo N, Sawamura S, Tanaka K, *et al.* The requirement of intestinal bacterial flora for the development of an IgE production system fully susceptible to oral tolerance induction. *J Immunol* 1997; 159:1739–1745.

26. Grönlund MM, Lehtonen OP, Eerola E, *et al.* Fecal microflora in healthy infants born by different methods of delivery: permanent changes in intestinal flora after cesarean delivery. *J Pediatr Gastroenterol Nutr* 1999; 28:19–25.

27. Grönlund MM, Arvilommi H, Kero P, *et al.* Importance of intestinal colonisation in the maturation of humoral immunity in early infancy: a prospective follow up study of healthy infants aged 0–6 months. *Arch Dis Child* 2000; 83:F186–192.

28. Sütas Y, Soppi E, Korhonen H, *et al.* Suppression of lymphocyte proliferation in vitro by bovine caseins hydrolysed with *Lactobacillus* GG-derived enzymes. *J Allergy Clin Immunol* 1996; 98:216–224.

29. Sütas Y, Hurme M, Isolauri E. Downregulation of antiCD3 antibody-induced IL-4 production by bovine caseins hydrolysed with *Lactobacillus* GG-derived enzymes. *Scand J Immunol* 1996; 43: 687–689.

30. Pessi T, Sütas Y, Hurme M, *et al.* Interleukin-10 generation in atopic children following

oral *Lactobacillus rhamnosus* GG. *Clin Exp Allergy* 2000; 30:1804–1808.

31. Kalliomäki M, Kirjavainen P, Eerola E, *et al.* Distinct patterns of neonatal gut microflora in infants in whom atopy was and was not developing . *J Allergy Clin Immunol* 2001; 107:129–134.

32. Kalliomäki M, Salminen S, Kero P, *et al.* Probiotics in the primary prevention of atopic disease: a randomised, placebo-controlled trial. *Lancet* 2001; 357:1076–1079.

33. Salminen S, von Wright A, Morelli L, *et al.* Demonstration of safety of probiotics – a review. *Int J Food Microbiol* 1998; 44:93–106.

34. MacFie J, O'Boyle C, Mitchell C, *et al.* Gut origin of sepsis: a prospective study investigating associations between bacterial translocation, gastric microflora, and septic morbidity. *Gut* 1999; 45:223–228.

35. Salminen S, von Wright A, Ouwehand AC, *et al.* Safety assessment of probiotics and starters. In: Adams M, Nout R, eds. *Fermentation and Food Safety.* Gaithersburg: Aspen Publishers, 2001: 239–325.

36. von Wright A, Sibakov M. Genetic modification of lactic acid bacteria. In: Salminen S, von Wright A, eds. *Lactic Acid Bacteria: Microbiology and functional aspects.* New York: Marcel Dekker, 1998: 161–210.

Inflammatory bowel disease: rationale for therapeutic focus on gut flora

Fergus Shanahan

14

Introduction: environmental factors in inflammatory bowel disease

The pathogenesis of both Crohn's disease and ulcerative colitis is complex and involves three interacting elements: genetic susceptibility factors, priming by the enteric microflora, and immune-mediated tissue injury.[1–3] Pathological intestinal inflammation appears to arise from abnormal immune reactivity to components of the intestinal microflora in genetically susceptible individuals. This conceptual model does not exclude a role for infectious agents as cofactors that condition mucosal immune responses and may determine the onset of disease. However, the process appears more complex than a simple struggle between microbe and human. Thus, infectious agents may exert their influence on inflammatory diseases by altering mucosal immune development, repertoire and cytokine profile, rather than simply mediating an infection of the target organ in a traditional sense.

Although there may be heterogeneity within Crohn's disease and ulcerative colitis, these two syndromes also have a curious relationship, being linked with genetic and environmental factors that are both shared and distinct.[4] Evidence for the impact of environmental factors in inflammatory bowel disease (IBD) includes:

- an incomplete concordance rate (<50% for Crohn's disease; <10% for ulcerative colitis) in monozygotic twins;
- variable rates in some ethnic groups living in different geographic locations;
- demonstrated effects of specific environmental factors such as smoking which influence severity and possibly phenotype;
- temporal changes in incidence and prevalence.

Epidemiological studies showing recent trends in IBD in different countries can only be explained by the action of environmental factors. The most reliable studies are population based, and these reveal increases in incidence and prevalence over recent decades as countries develop and become industrialised.[5,6]

In the wake of the somewhat sobering lesson of *Helicobacter pylori* and peptic disease, many clinicians are perhaps excessively cautious and too ready to adopt an infection-oriented concept for the pathogenesis of all 'idiopathic' disorders.[7] Certainly, an infectious basis would be a conceptually appealing explanation for recent trends in the prevalence of IBD. However, although the action of an environmental factor(s) is indisputable, it does not necessarily imply a transmissible agent: there are other potential mechanisms for an environmental impact. It is noteworthy that trends in prevalence of IBD have not occurred in isolation: they parallel similar increases in the prevalence of several other conditions including allergies, asthma, multiple sclerosis and insulin-dependent diabetes mellitus.[8,9] These are all immunologically mediated disorders, and it seems likely that environmental factors are exerting their effects via the immune system rather than mediating transmissible infections of different target organs.

The immune system is a sensory organ designed for interpreting the environment, alerting the host to danger and eliminating danger when it enters the internal milieu. As with other senses, development and learning require sensory input or education. Reduced or altered immunologic sensory input leads to disturbed immune regulation and might account for the apparent rise in immunologically mediated disorders. In this respect, environmental contact with childhood infections and commensal flora is responsible for the fine-tuning of T-cell repertoires and cytokine balance within the gut mucosa.[9] Contributory elements of the modern lifestyle in industrialised societies that affect immune development include changes in sanitation, hygiene, antibiotic usage, life on concrete with reduced exposure to soil microorganisms, consumption of sterile food and beverages, non-fermented foods and vaccination. Indeed, conditions that would promote the transmission of a pathogenic infection, such as overcrowding, poor sanitation and endemic parasitism, actually appear to protect against IBD![10,11]

Small talk within the gut

The local microenvironment and mucosal integrity

Given the impact of commensal flora on mucosal immune development and defence,[9,12] it is appropriate to examine the importance of the flora in mucosal homeostasis. The gastrointestinal lumen is a dynamic open ecosystem in continuity with the external environment. Its content of microflora comprises 10 times more bacteria than cells in the human body, over 400 bacterial species, and accounts for approximately 1–2 kg body weight.[13–16] The metabolic activity of this 'neglected organ' is poorly understood, but may rival that of the liver. Under normal circumstances the microflora is an asset,[12] but, depending on environmental conditions and host susceptibility, it may become a liability and the distinction between a pathogen and a commensal becomes less clear. At least 50% of the bacterial composition of the human gut flora is 'unculturable' at present, but it is

identifiable by molecular methods. Such studies have confirmed the bacterial diversity within humans, which appears to be both individual and stable in adults over time.[17,18]

The impact of the environment on the flora and the role of the flora in defence are illustrated by the overgrowth of opportunistic organisms, such as *Clostridium difficile,* in some individuals following antibiotic usage. Host genetics also affect the composition of the flora, and this may have particular relevance to IBD.[18, 19]

The conditioning effects of the normal bacterial flora on structure and function have been known for decades from seminal observations in germ-free animals.[16] The presence of bacteria within the lumen influences epithelial turnover, smooth muscle function and motility, local endocrine activity, intestinal vascularity and mucosal immune development and function. The microflora, therefore, exchanges regulatory signals with the epithelial and subepithelial components of the intestine.[20,21] The molecular basis for the multidirectional host–flora interactions is now being studied using multiple gene expression analysis. The bacterial signals are not well understood but include formylated peptides, bacterial nucleotides, lipopolysaccharide (LPS), peptidoglycans and other bacterial cell wall constituents.

In addition to educating the mucosal immune response, the bacterial flora prime and maintain it in a state of restrained immune reactivity, in ready alert for the episodic threat of pathogenic challenge. Therefore, the normal mucosa is in a state of 'controlled (physiologic) inflammation'. This requires exquisitely precise control. One level of control involves the network of intercellular connectivities within the intestine that includes not only signals to and from the flora, but also lymphoepithelial dialogue, and neuroimmune and stromal interactions.[22] Another level of control is the presence of regulatory T cells within the intestinal mucosa, which has been demonstrated in studies of animal models where lymphocyte subpopulations are transferred to immune-deficient animals.[23,24] It appears that regulatory T cells control immune reactivity to enteric bacteria and keep physiologic inflammation within the mucosa in check. Failure of this regulation enables progression to pathologic inflammation. Regulatory T cells within the intestine appear to be similar to peripheral T-cell subpopulations responsible for preventing autoimmunity to tissue-specific self-antigens. Local immunosuppression by these cells is mediated by the production of IL-10 and TGF-β, and is dependent on signalling via the cytotoxic T lymphocyte-associated antigen 4 (CTLA-4), which is a negative regulator of T-cell activation.[25] In addition, control of immune and inflammatory events requires an ability to turn off immune responses once offending pathogens have been dealt with. This is normally achieved by induction of apoptosis within activated lymphocytes, a process that appears defective in Crohn's disease and results in the accumulation of activated T cells within lesions.[26–28]

Sampling the microbial environment within the gut

As with other sensory systems, the mucosal immune system samples the environment with sensory (antigen) receptors, relays information along afferent and efferent limbs, and exhibits memory, learning and adaptation.[22] Sampling of antigens from the lumen occurs across specialised M cells overlying lymphoid follicles[29] and across the columnar epithelium.[30,31] In both cases, antigens are delivered to dendritic cells which function as antigen-presenting cells (APC) for the initiation of immune responses. There is evidence for tissue-specific specialisation of intestinal dendritic cells that determines the pattern of cytokines produced and differentiation of T cells (Th1 or Th2) after exposure to antigens.[32] In addition to transepithelial and interepithelial antigen sampling from the lumen, columnar enterocytes also have a sensory function.[33] Enterocytes alert the host to a breach in the mucosal barrier by invasive pathogens and direct the immune response to the site of entry. This is achieved by temporal and spatial production of a range of chemokines and cytokines.[33,34] The signal transduction pathway for cytokine production by enterocytes involves the transcription factor NFκB, and it has been shown that non-pathogenic components of the flora may attenuate proinflammatory responses by blocking degradation of the counterregulatory factor IκB.[35] This points to a critical difference between pathogenic and non-pathogenic bacteria within the gut, and may provide useful insights into the mode of action of probiotics.

Discrimination of harmless commensals from dangerous pathogens is mediated, at least in part, by pattern recognition receptors or Toll-like receptors (TLRs). These are expressed on epithelial cells and on antigen-presenting cells.[36] Altered expression of TLRs is evident in IBD,[37] and one might predict that some of the genes associated with IBD will be linked with polymorphisms in the molecular recognition of luminal bacteria by such receptors.

The intestinal flora in IBD

Alterations in gut flora have been described in patients with inflammatory bowel disease but findings have been inconsistent.[1,12] Enteroadherent strains of *Escherichia coli* in the ileal mucosa have been found in patients with Crohn's disease.[38] More recently, a novel bacterial sequence has been reported in association with intestinal lesions in patients

with Crohn's disease.[39] These observations may be secondary to the disease process rather than a primary event. One pathogen that is often proposed as the cause of Crohn's disease is *Mycobacterium paratuberculosis*. However, infections with intracellular pathogens are difficult to reconcile with the remarkable efficacy of anti-TNF-α therapy that can produce complete mucosal healing for prolonged periods by repeated infusion.[40] Antagonism of TNF-α has been sufficient to be a risk for active *M. tuberculosis* infection, yet disseminated *M. paratuberculosis* has not been reported in this setting.

Although one cannot exclude a role for pathogenic organisms, persuasive evidence indicates that normal enteric bacterial flora drive the inflammatory process in IBD.

1. The lesions occur in areas of the bowel with the highest bacterial counts.

2. Diversion of the faecal stream in Crohn's disease has a beneficial effect on distal disease and recurrence is predictable after restoration of the continuity of the stream.[41–44]

3. The relationship between disease recurrence and direct contact with luminal contents has been demonstrated directly.[45–47]

4. The occurrence of pouchitis in patients with pre-existing ulcerative colitis, but not in those with familial polyposis, and its response to antibiotics, indicates a role

of the bacterial flora in this human disease 'model' that is dependent on the genetic constitution of the host.

5. Studies of lymphocyte responsiveness to autologous and heterologous intestinal bacteria have indicated a loss of immunological tolerance to the enteric flora in patients with active inflammatory bowel disease and in experimental models of enterocolitis.[48–50] This is reflected by serologic reactivity to enteric bacteria,[51] and cross-reactivity between autoantibodies such as antineutrophil cytoplasmic antibodies (ANCA) and enteric bacterial antigens.[52]

6. Colonisation with intestinal bacteria is required for expression of the inflammatory disease in animal models of IBD, irrespective of the underlying genetic defect.[53–55]

7. In animal models, IBD has been transferred with effector T cells reactive against enteric bacteria.[56]

A limited number of bacterial antigens appear to be responsible for driving the inflammatory response.[56] Furthermore, enteric bacteria vary in their capacity to drive intestinal inflammation. *Lactobacillus* and *Bifidobacterium* species have no apparent proinflammatory capacity and have been used as probiotics. In contrast, other bacteria, such as *Bacteroides vulgatus,* can cause colitis when monoassociated in the HLA-B27 transgenic

rat model.[57] Other organisms, such as *Helicobacter hepaticus,* have been reported to cause colitis in pathogen-free severe combined immunodeficient (*scid*) and IL-10-deficient mice, but not in controls.[58]

Ecotherapeutics – the promise of probiotics in IBD

With the exception of antibiotics, conventional drug therapy for IBD is directed toward suppression or modulation of the immunoinflammatory response. Until recently, little attention has been devoted to the microenvironment as a therapeutic opportunity. Probiotics are viable microorganisms that have a beneficial effect on health by altering the commensal flora. *Prebiotics* are dietary substances, usually polysaccharide in nature, that also favourably alter the enteric flora, and *synbiotics* are combinations of probiotics and prebiotics. Probiotic bacteria are frequently members of the genera lactobacillus and bifidobacterium, but *E. coli,* enterococci and non-bacterial species, such as *Saccharomyces boulardii,* have been used as probiotics. Although many of the claims for probiotic efficacy have not been evidence based,[59,60] well-designed trials have demonstrated the beneficial impact of probiotics in infectious diseases.[61,62]

The impact of probiotic therapy on different animal models of IBD has been confirmed by several investigators.[63] In addition to apparent anti-inflammatory effects, a strain of *L. salivarius* (*ssp salivarius UCC118*) diminished the rate of progression from inflammation through dysplasia to colon cancer in IL-10-deficient mice, compared with non-probiotic-fed animals.[64,65] Several mechanisms for an anticancer effect have been proposed for probiotics, particularly in relation to colon cancer.[66] In humans, a non-pathogenic strain of *E. coli* has been reported to have efficacy equivalent to that of mesalazine in patients with ulcerative colitis.[67,68] Perhaps the most impressive evidence for efficacy of probiotics in IBD has been the maintenance of remission of patients with pouchitis using a cocktail of eight bacterial strains.[69] As with drug combinations, it is desirable that the properties of the individual components are well characterised before routine use. In this respect, our group has developed probiotic strains that can be identified and recovered in stool, and for which the sequencing of the bacterial genome will be completed soon[65,70,71] (and unpublished observations).

More recently, the introduction of organisms genetically engineered to produce and deliver anti-inflammatory cytokines or other biologically relevant molecules to the inflamed mucosa promises to extend the scope and potential of probiotic action.[72,73] Proof of principle with this technique has been achieved with a food-grade *Lactococcus lactis*

engineered to secrete IL-10 within the gut. The therapeutic efficacy of this strategy was shown in two murine experimental models of IBD.[72] However, safety concerns must be overcome before this therapeutic approach can be applied to humans, but obvious advantages will include cost-effectiveness, convenience of delivery and organ specificity.

Conclusion

Compelling evidence, albeit circumstantial, has implicated the gut flora in the pathogenesis of IBD. Although current therapeutic strategies are largely limited to suppression of the host response, manipulation of the microenvironment by altering the intestinal microflora is emerging as a realistic therapeutic strategy. The mechanism of action of probiotics is unclear: their action in infectious disease may differ from that in inflammatory disease. In the latter process it seems likely that signalling with the epithelium is involved, as occurs normally with some of the resident flora. However, enthusiasm for probiotic therapy should be tempered by several caveats. Much work needs to be done to clarify optimal dosages, frequency of administration, delivery vehicle and optimal choice of strain. In addition, it cannot be assumed that a single probiotic will be suited to all patients, or indeed to all stages of the same disease. Well-designed controlled trials in IBD are required to bring probiotic therapy into the arena of evidence-based medicine. More importantly, an improved understanding of the normal flora is required before the true value of probiotics and other forms of therapeutic modulation of the flora can be fully realised.

Acknowledgement

The author's work is supported in part by the Health Research Board of Ireland, the Higher Education Authority of Ireland and the European Union (PROGID: QLK1-2000-00563).

References

1. Sartor RB. Enteric microflora in IBD: pathogens or commensals? *Inflamm Bowel Dis* 1997; 3:230–235.

2. Shanahan F. Inflammatory bowel disease: immunodiagnostics, immunotherapeutics and ecotherapeutics. *Gastroenterology* 2001; 120: 622–635.

3. Elson CO. Commensal bacteria as targets in Crohn's disease. *Gastroenterology* 2000; 119: 254–257.

4. Taylor KD, Rotter JI, Yang H. Genetics of inflammatory bowel disease. In: Targan SR, Shanahan F, Karp LC, eds. *Inflammatory Bowel Disease: From Bench to Bedside* 2nd edn. Dordrecht: Kluwer Academic, 2001.

5. Loftus EV Jr, Silverstein MD, Sandborn WJ, Tremaine WJ, Harmsen WS, Zinsmeister AR. Crohn's disease in Olmsted County, Minnesota, 1940–1993: incidence, prevalence, and survival. *Gastroenterology* 1998; 114:1161–1168.

6. Bernstein CN, Blanchard JF, Rawsthorne P, Wajda A. Epidemiology of Crohn's disease and ulcerative colitis in a central Canadian province: a population-based study. *Am J Epidemiol* 1999; 149:916–924.

7. Lorber B. Are all diseases infectious? *Ann Intern Med* 1996; 125:844–851.

8. Herz U, Lacy P, Renz H, Erb K. The influence of infections on the development and severity of allergic disorders. *Curr Opin Immunol* 2000; 12:632–640.

9. Rook GA, Stanford JL. Give us this day our daily germs. *Immunol Today* 1998; 19: 113–116.

10. Gent AE, Hellier MD, Grace RH, Swarbrick ET, Coggon D. Inflammatory bowel disease and domestic hygiene in infancy. *Lancet* 1994; 343:766–767.

11. Elliott DE, Urban JF Jr., Argo CK, Weinstock JV. Does the failure to acquire helminthic parasites predispose to Crohn's disease? *FASEB J* 2000; 14:1848–1855.

12. Shanahan F. Probiotics and inflammatory bowel disease: is there a scientific rationale? *Inflamm Bowel Dis* 2000; 6:107–115.

13. Bocci V. The neglected organ: bacterial flora has a crucial immunostimulatory role. *Perspect Biol Med* 1992; 35:251–260.

14. Mackowiak PA. The normal microbial flora. *N Engl J Med* 1982; 307:83–93.

15. Berg RD. The indigenous gastrointestinal microflora. *Trends Microbiol* 1996; 4: 430–435.

16. Midtvedt T. Microbial functional activities. In: Hanson LA, Yolken RH, eds. *Intestinal*

Microflora. Nestlè Nutrition Workshop Series. Philadelphia: Lippincott-Raven, 1999; 42: 79–96.

17. Vaughan EE, Schut F, Heilig HGHJ, Zoetendal EG, de Vos WM, Akkermans ADL. A molecular view of the intestinal ecosystem. *Curr Issues Intest Microbiol* 2000; 1:1–12.

18. Akkermans ADL, Zoetendal EG, Favier CF, Heilig HGHJ, Akkermans-van Vliet WM, de Vos WM. Temperature and denaturing gradient gel electrophoresis analysis of 16S rRNA from human faecal samples. *Biosci Microflora* 2000; 19:93–98.

19. Van de Merwe JP, Stegeman JH, Hazenberg MP. The resident faecal flora is determined by genetic characteristics of the host. Implications for Crohn's disease? *Antonie van Leeuwenhoek* 1983; 49:119–124.

20. Gordon JI, Hooper LV, McNevin SM, Wong M, Bry L. Epithelial cell growth and differentiation III. Promoting diversity in the intestine: conversations between the microflora, epithelium, and diffuse GALT. *Am J Physiol* 1997; 273: G565–G570.

21. Bry L, Falk PG, Midtvedt T, Gordon JI. A model system of host-microbial interactions in an open mammalian ecosystem. *Science* 1996; 273:1380–1383.

22. Shanahan F. Mechanisms of immunologic sensation of intestinal contents. *Am J Physiol* 2000; 278:G191–G196.

23. Powrie F. T cells in inflammatory bowel disease: protective and pathogenic roles. *Immunity* 1995; 3:171–174.

24. Kronenberg M, Cheroutre H. Do mucosal T cells prevent intestinal inflammation? *Gastroenterology* 2000; 118:974–977.

25. Read S, Malmström V, Powrie F. Cytotoxic T lymphocyte-associated antigen 4 plays an essential role in the function of CD25+CD4+ regulatory cells that control intestinal inflammation. *J Exp Med* 2000; 192:295–302.

26. Boirivant M, Marini M, Di Felice G, *et al.* Lamina propria T cells in Crohn's disease and other gastrointestinal inflammation show defective CD2 pathway-induced apoptosis. *Gastroenterology* 1999; 116:557–565.

27. Ina K, Itoh J, Fukushima K, Kusugami K, *et al.* Resistance of Crohn's disease T cells to multiple apoptotic signals is associated with a Bcl-2/Bax mucosal imbalance. *J Immunol* 1999; 163:1081–1090.

28. Atreya R, Mudter J, Finotto S, *et al.* Blockade of interleukin 6 *trans* signalling suppresses T-cell resistance against apoptosis in chronic intestinal inflammation: evidence in Crohn's disease and experimental colitis *in vivo*. *Nature Med* 2000; 6:583–588.

29. Neutra MR. Role of M cells in transepithelial transport of antigens and pathogens to the mucosal immune system. *Am J Physiol Gastrointest Liver Physiol* 1998; 274: G785–G791.

30. Gewirtz AT, Madara JL. Periscope, up! Monitoring microbes in the intestine. *Nature Immunol* 2001; 2:288–290.

31. Rescigno M, Urbano M, Valzasina B, *et al.* Dendritic cells express tight junction proteins and penetrate gut epithelial monolayers to sample bacteria. *Nature Immunol* 2001; 2: 361–367.

32. Iwasaki A, Kelsall BL. Freshly isolated Peyer's patch but not spleen, dendritic cells produce interleukin 10 and induce the differentiation of T helper type 2 cells. *J Exp Med* 1999; 190: 229–239.

33. Kagnoff MF, Eckmann L. Epithelial cells as

sensors for microbial infection. *J Clin Invest* 1997; 100:6–10.

34. Luster AD. Chemokines regulate lymphocyte homing to the intestinal mucosa. *Gastroenterology* 2001; 120:291–294.

35. Neish AS, Gewirtz AT, Zeng H, *et al.* Prokaryotic regulation of epithelial responses by inhibition of IκB-α ubiquitination. *Science* 2000; 289:1560–1563.

36. Cario E, Rosenberg IM, Brandwein SL, Beck PL, Reinecker H-C, Podolsky DK. Lipopolysaccharide activates distinct signalling pathways in intestinal epithelial cell lines expressing Toll-like receptors. *J Immunol* 2000; 164:966–972.

37. Cario E, Podolsky DK. Differential alteration in intestinal epithelial cell expression of toll-like receptor 3 (TLR3) and TLR4 in inflammatory bowel disease. *Infect Immun* 2000; 68:7010–7017.

38. Darfeuille-Michaud A, Neut C, Barnich N, *et al.* Presence of adherent *Escherichia coli* strains in ileal mucosa of patients with Crohn's disease. *Gastroenterology* 1998; 115: 1405–1413.

39. Sutton CL, Kim J, Yamane A, *et al.* Identification of a novel bacterial sequence associated with Crohn's disease. *Gastroenterology* 2000; 119:23–31.

40. Rutgeerts P, D'Haens G, Targan S, *et al.* Efficacy and safety of retreatment with anti-tumor necrosis factor antibody (infliximab) to maintain remission in Crohn's disease. *Gastroenterology* 1999; 117:761–769.

41. Janowitz HD, Croen EC, Sacher DB. The role of the fecal stream in Crohn's disease: an historical and analytical review. *Inflamm Bowel Dis* 1998; 4:29–39.

42. Rutgeerts P, Geboes K, Peeters M, *et al.* Effect of faecal stream diversion on recurrence of Crohn's disease in the neoterminal ileum. *Lancet* 1991; 338:771–774.

43. Rutgeerts P, Geboes K, Vantrappen G, Beyls J, Kerremans R, Hiele M. Predictability of the postoperative course of Crohn's disease. *Gastroenterology* 1990; 99:956–963.

44. Tytgat GNJ, Mulder CJJ, Brummelkamp WH. Endoscopic lesions in Crohn's disease early after ileocecal resection. *Endoscopy* 1988; 20:260–262.

45. Harper PH, Lee ECG, Kettlewell MGW, Bennett MK, Jewell DP. Role of the faecal stream in the maintenance of Crohn's colitis. *Gut* 1985; 26:279–284.

46. D'Haens GR, Geboes K, Peeters M, Baert F, Penninckx F, Rutgeerts P. Early lesions of recurrent Crohn's disease caused by infusion of intestinal contents in excluded ileum. *Gastroenterology* 1998; 114:262–267.

47. Sartor RB. Postoperative recurrence of Crohn's disease: the enemy is within the fecal stream. *Gastroenterology* 1998; 114:398–407.

48. Duchmann R, Kaiser I, Hermann E, Mayet W, Ewe K, Meyer zum Büschenfelde K-H. Tolerance exists towards resident intestinal flora but is broken in active inflammatory bowel disease (IBD). *Clin Exp Immunol* 1995; 102:448–455.

49. Duchmann R, Schmitt E, Knolle P, Meyer zum Büschenfelde K-H, Neurath M. Tolerance towards resident intestinal flora in mice is abrogated in experimental colitis and restored by treatment with interleukin-10 or antibodies to interleukin-12. *Eur J Immunol* 1996; 26:934–938.

50. Duchmann R, May E, Heike M, Knolle P, Neurath M, Meyer zum Büschenfelde K-H. T cell specificity and cross reactivity toward

enterobacteria, *Bacteroides, Bifidobacterium,* and antigens from resident intestinal flora in humans. *Gut* 1999; 44:812–818.

51. MacPherson A, Khoo UY, Forgacs I, Philpott-Howard J, Bjarnason I. Mucosal antibodies in inflammatory bowel disease are directed against intestinal bacteria. *Gut* 1996; 38: 365–375.

52. Shanahan F. Immunologic and genetic links in Crohn's disease. *Gut* 2000; 46:6–7.

53. Elson CO, Sartor RB, Tennyson GS, Riddell RH. Experimental models of inflammatory bowel disease. *Gastroenterology* 1995; 109: 1344–1367.

54. Fuss IJ, Strober W. Animal models of inflammatory bowel disease: insights into the immunopathogenesis of Crohn's disease and ulcerative colitis. *Curr Opin Gastroenterol* 1998; 14:476–482.

55. Blumberg RS, Saubermann LJ, Strober W. Animal models of mucosal inflammation and their relation to human inflammatory bowel disease. *Curr Opin Immunol* 1999; 11: 648–656.

56. Cong Y, Brandwein SL, McCabe RP, *et al.* CD4+ T cells reactive to enteric bacterial antigens in spontaneously colitic C3H/HeJBir mice: increased T helper cell type 1 response and ability to transfer disease. *J Exp Med* 1998; 187:855–864.

57. Rath HC, Herfarth HH, Ikeda JS, *et al.* Normal luminal bacteria, especially *Bacteroides* species, mediate chronic colitis, gastritis, and arthritis in HLA-B27/human beta 2 microglobulin transgenic rats. *J Clin Invest* 1996; 98:945–953.

58. Kulberg MC, Ward MJ, Gorelick PL, *et al.* *Helicobacter hepaticus* triggers colitis in specific pathogen-free interleukin-10 (IL-10)-deficient mice through an IL-12- and gamma-interferon-dependent mechanism. *Infect Immun* 1998; 66:5157–5166.

59. Berg RD. Probiotics, prebiotics or 'conbiotics'? *Trends Microbiol* 1998; 6:89–92.

60. Atlas RM. Probiotics – snake oil for the new millenium? Environmental *Microbiol* 1999; 1:375–382.

61. Surawicz CM, McFarland LV, Elmer GW, *et al.* Treatment of recurrent *Clostridium difficile* colitis with vancomycin and *Saccharomyces boulardii. Am J Gastroenterol* 1989; 84: 1285–1287.

62. Vanderhoof JA, Whitney DB, Antonson DL, *et al. Lactobacillus GG* in the prevention of antibiotic-associated diarrhea in children. *J Pediatr* 1999; 135:564–568.

63. Madsen KL, Doyle JS, Jewell LD, Tavernini MM, Fedorak RN. *Lactobacillus* species prevents colitis in interleukin 10 gene-deficient mice. *Gastroenterology* 1999; 116: 1107–1114.

64. Collins JK, Murphy L, O'Mahony L, Dunne C, O'Sullivan GC, Shanahan F. A controlled trial of probiotic treatment of IL-10 knockout mice. *Gastroenterology* 1999; 116:G2981.

65. O'Mahony L, Feeney M, O'Halloran S, *et al.* Probiotic impact on microbial flora inflammation and tumor development in IL-10 knock out mice. *Aliment Pharmacol Ther* 2001; 15:1219–1225.

66. Dugas B, Mercenier A, Lenoir-Wijnkoop I, Arnaud C, Dugas N, Postaire E. Immunity and probiotics. *Immunol Today* 1999; 20: 387–390.

67. Kruis W, Schütz E, Fric P, Fixa B, Judmaiers G, Stolte M. Double-blind comparison of an oral *Escherichia coli* preparation and mesalazine in maintaining remission of

ulcerative colitis. *Aliment Pharmacol Ther* 1997; 11:853–858.

68. Rembacken BJ, Snelling AM, Hawkey PM, Chalmers DM, Axon ATR. Non-pathogenic *Escherichia coli* versus mesalazine for the treatment of ulcerative colitis: a randomised trial. *Lancet* 1999; 354:635–639.

69. Gionchietti P, Rizzello F, Venturi A, *et al*. Oral bacteriotherapy as maintenance treatment in patients with chronic pouchitis: a double blind, placebo-controlled trial. *Gastroenterology* 2000; 119:305–309.

70. Dunne C, Murphy L, Flynn S, *et al*. Probiotics: from myth to reality. Demonstration of functionality in animal models of disease and in human clinical trials. *Antonie von Leeuwenhoek* 1999; 76:279–292.

71. Murphy L, Dunne C, Kiely B, Shanahan F, O'Sullivan GC, Collins JK. In vivo assessment of potential probiotic *Lactobacillus salivarius* strains: evaluation of their establishment, persistence, and localisation in the murine gastrointestinal tract. *Microb Ecol Health Dis* 1999; 11:149–157.

72. Steidler L, Hans W, Schotte L, *et al*. Treatment of murine colitis by *Lactococcus lactis* secreting interleukin-10. *Science* 2000; 289:1352–1355.

73. Shanahan F. Therapeutic manipulation of gut flora. *Science* 2000; 289:1311–1312.

Inflammatory bowel disease and probiotics

Paolo Gionchetti, Fernando Rizzello and Massimo Campieri

15

Introduction

The gastrointestinal tract, with an approximate surface area similar to that of a tennis court (200–250 m²), and the respiratory system, with an approximate surface area similar to that of a soccer field, represent the largest mucosal surfaces connecting the human body with the environment. The gastrointestinal mucosal surface, in spite of its small area compared with the lung, has more complex functions. In fact, the gastrointestinal tract can be regarded as a reservoir with an internal surface separating 10^{13} eukaryotic cells from 10^{14} bacterial cells.[1]

The colonisation of the alimentary tract begins immediately after birth. The bacterial distribution pattern and concentration vary greatly at different levels of the gastrointestinal tract, ranging from $< 10^3$ CFU/ml (colony forming unit/ml) in the stomach, where the number of the ingested bacteria is dramatically reduced by contact with gastric acid, to 10^{11}–10^{12} CFU/ml within the colon, where anaerobes outnumber aerobes by a ratio of 1000:1. Along the length of the small intestine there is a transition to a higher concentration of bacteria and an increasing predominance of

Gram-negative species in the distal ileum, with a dramatic increase in bacterial concentration across the ileocaecal valve. The complexity of resident colonic flora is illustrated by the presence of more than 400 bacterial species. These viable bacteria represent one-third of faecal dry weight.[2]

The presence of the indigenous flora is important for the maturation of the immune system and for the development of normal intestinal morphology. The gut represents a complex ecosystem in which the intestinal microflora and the host interact in order to maintain a chronic immunologically balanced intestinal inflammatory response ('physiologic inflammation'). The host has acquired various protective defence mechanisms to maintain this delicate balance:

- the barrier provided by the epithelial layer;
- mechanical factors, such as peristalsis and desquamation;
- factors that interfere with bacterial attachment, such as the mucous layer and secretory immunoglobulin A (IgA), which represent the primary immune barrier against pathogens.

At the beginning of the 20th century the Russian Nobel Prize Laureate Elie Metchnikoff first made the hypothesis that a high concentration of lactobacilli in the composition of the intestinal flora could be very important for the preservation of health and the achievement of longevity.[3] At the same time Tissier[4] showed that bifidobacteria were the predominant intestinal microbial flora in breastfed infants. This consideration supported the speculation that infant diarrhoea could be treated with large doses of bifidobacteria.

Lilly and Stilwell introduced the term 'probiotic' in 1965, to describe any substance or organism that contributes to intestinal microbial balance.[5] Fuller[6] subsequently modified this definition by stressing the crucial importance of a live microbial feed supplement. More recently, probiotics have been defined as 'living organisms, which upon ingestion in certain numbers, exert health benefits beyond inherent basic nutrition',[7] emphasising the importance of maintaining a sufficient population of live microorganisms in the gut and further implying that benefits, such as improvement in microbial balance, may also be associated with other effects, such as immunomodulation.

Most probiotics belong to a large group designated lactic acid bacteria, because lactic acid is the major end-product of their metabolism. This group includes lactobacilli, streptococci and bifidobacteria. New probiotics may include other types of bacteria, such as *Clostridium* and *Bacillus subtilis,* and even non-bacterial organisms such as *Saccharomyces boulardii.* Probiotic strains must possess some necessary characteristics (Table 15.1):

Table 15.1
Desirable properties of probiotic bacteria

- *Human origin*
- *Resistance to acid and bile*
- *Ability to sustain metabolic activity within the gut lumen*
- *Ability transiently to colonise the human gut*
- *Antagonism against pathogenic bacteria*
- *Safe for human use*
- *Clinically validated health effects*
- *Ability to maintain viability and other beneficial properties through processing, culture and storage*

- They must be normal inhabitants of the intestinal tract and of human origin, because some health-promoting effects may be species specific.
- They need to be able to survive the acid of the stomach, the digestive enzymes and bile salts.
- They must have the ability to be metabolically active within the luminal flora, where ideally they should survive, if not persist, in the long term.
- They must be safe for human use and should maintain their viability and beneficial properties through processing, culture and storage.[8]

The 'probiotic concept' is still controversial, because the beneficial effects have been shown mainly under experimental conditions, and because the precise mechanisms by which probiotic microorganisms exert their effect on the host *in vivo* are poorly defined. Supposed mechanisms of action include:

1. colonisation resistance: a complex of actions, including the production of antimicrobial substances such as bacteriocin, competition for nutrients, competition for receptors and reduction of luminal colonic pH, in order to antagonise pathogenic bacteria;

2. promotion of a non-specific stimulation of the host immune system, including immune cell proliferation, enhanced phagocytic activity and increased production of secretory IgA, and indeed Wagner *et al.*[9] have demonstrated that the systemic dissemination of *Candida albicans* decreases, with a consequent reduction in mortality, if four different probiotic strains (*Lactobacillus acidophilus, Lactobacillus GG, Lactobacillus reuterii* and *Bifidobacterium animalis*) are given to congenitally immune-deficient mice;[9]

3. production of nutrients such as short-chain fatty acids (SCFA) and vitamins;

4. removal of toxic substances.

Probiotics in inflammatory bowel disease

Despite the progress that has been made in

the detection of the pathogenetic mechanism, the aetiology of inflammatory bowel disease (IBD) remains unclear. A specific pathogen associated with these diseases has not been found. On the contrary, there is an increasing number of both clinical and experimental data that suggest a central role for the gut flora in driving the inflammatory responses in these disorders.[10] The areas with the highest luminal bacterial concentration are the distal ileum and the colon, which also represent the sites most frequently affected by inflammation in patients with IBD.[11] Similarly, pouchitis, the non-specific inflammation frequently present in the ileal reservoir after ileoanal anastomosis, develops in the presence of bacterial overgrowth. Enteric bacteria or their phlogistic products have been detected within the inflamed mucosa of patients with Crohn's disease. The evidence of a breakdown of normal tolerance to the commensal flora in active IBD[12,13] suggests that the hyperreactivity to ubiquitous antigens from the enteric microflora is implicated at least in the perpetuation of inflammation. In patients with Crohn's disease, it is well known that antibiotics or faecal stream diversion can reduce disease activity, with disease recurrence occurring after restoration of the stream.[14] In addition, antibiotics are the first choice of therapy in pouchitis. Recent studies have shown the ability of the ileostomy effluent – presumably dominated by bacteria or their products – of Crohn's disease patients to trigger postoperative recurrence in the excluded normal ileal loop of the same patient within a few days.[15] Finally, purified bacterial products are able to initiate and perpetuate experimental colitis in many transgenic and knockout murine models of colitis, but the inflammation is not seen when these animals are maintained in germ-free conditions.[16]

These observations suggest that the gut inflammation may be associated with an imbalance in the intestinal microflora, with a relative predominance of 'aggressive' bacteria and an insufficient concentration of 'protective' species. A possible therapeutic strategy in IBD may involve manipulation of the local microenvironment, in order to restore the microbial balance.[17]

There is increasing evidence that probiotics may play a role in the treatment of IBD. A significant reduction in lactobacillus concentration has been found in colonic biopsy specimens obtained from patients with active ulcerative colitis (UC)[18] and a decrease in bifidobacteria and lactobacilli has been reported in patients with Crohn's disease.[19] In addition, reduced faecal concentrations of bifidobacteria have been reported in pouchitis.[20] The administration of different strains of lactobacilli has shown beneficial effects in several animal models of experimental colitis. In particular, exogenous administration of *Lactobacillus reuterii*, either as pure bacterial suspension or as fermented oatmeal soup, was effective in ameliorating acetic acid-induced colitis[21] or methotrexate-induced colitis[22] in rats. More recently, *Lactobacillus* sp. was shown to be able to prevent the development of spontaneous colitis in interleukin-10 (IL-10)-deficient mice,[23] and continuous feeding with *Lactobacillus plantarum* was able to attenuate an established colitis in the same knockout model.[24] With regard to human data, the efficacy of a non-pathogenic strain of *Escherichia coli* (Nissle 1917) in the treatment of IBD has been tested in three recent trials. In the first pilot study the treatment with capsules containing *E. coli* Nissle 1917 was compared to the administration of placebo in the maintenance of steroid-induced remission of colonic Crohn's disease. At the end of the 12-week treatment period, relapse rates were 33% in the *E. coli* group and 63% in the placebo group. Unfortunately, because of the very small number of patients treated, this difference did not reach statistical significance.[25] In the other two controlled studies, patients with UC in remission were given oral mesalamine or *E. coli* Nissle 1917 as maintenance treatment. No significant difference in the relapse rate was shown between the two treatments. However, the first study had a short follow-up period,[26] and in the second study,[27] in our opinion, the low dose of mesalamine administered in the follow-up and the very high relapse rate (about 70%) in both groups limit the value of the findings.

In a small comparative controlled trial, Guslandi *et al.*[28] have evaluated the efficacy of *Saccharomyces boulardii* in maintenance treatment of Crohn's disease. Thirty-two patients with Crohn's disease in remission were randomised to receive either mesalamine 3 g/day or a combination of mesalamine (2 g/day) and *Saccharomyces boulardii* (1 g/day) for 6 months. A clinical relapse was observed in 37% of patients receiving mesalamine alone, and in 6.2% of patients treated receiving the combined treatment.

We adopted a different strategy using a new oral probiotic preparation, VSL#3, which is characterised by a very high bacterial concentration and by the presence of a cocktail of eight different bacterial species with potential synergistic relations (Table 15.2). This product contains 300 billion/g of viable lyophilised bacteria of four strains of lactobacilli (*L. casei*, *L. plantarum*, *L. acidophilus*, *L. delbrueckii* subsp. *bulgaricus*), three strains of bifidobacteria (*B. longum*,

Table 15.2
Composition of VSL#3

*300 billion viable lyophilised bacteria/g of four strains of lactobacilli (*L. casei, L. plantarum, L. acidophilus *and* L. delbrueckii *subsp.* bulgaricus*), three strains of bifidobacteria (*B. longum, B. breve *and* B. infantis*) and one strain of* Streptococcus salivarius *subsp.* thermophilus

B. breve, B. infantis) and one strain of *Streptococcus salivarius* subspecies *thermophilus*. A composite mixture of a large number of different strains may represent the optimal treatment, in view of the different and specialised metabolic activities of different probiotic organisms and the heterogeneity of the diseases. Initially, we obtained encouraging results in a pilot study using VSL#3 as maintenance treatment in 20 patients with UC in clinical, endoscopic and histological remission. These patients, who were allergic to mesalamine and sulphasalazine, received 6 g/day of VSL#3 for 1 year. At defined intervals they were assessed clinically and endoscopically, and samples for stool culture and determination of faecal pH were obtained. A significant increase in concentration of lactobacilli, bifidobacteria and *Streptococcus salivarius* subspecies *thermophilus* was evident after few days of treatment and persisted throughout the period of the study. The effective alteration in microbial intestinal flora composition was confirmed by a significant reduction of faecal pH. At the end of the study, 15 of 20 treated patients (75%) were still in remission.[29]

Subsequently, we evaluated the efficacy of the same probiotic preparation versus placebo in maintenance treatment of chronic pouchitis. Pouchitis, a non-specific inflammation of the ileal reservoir, is the major long-term complication following ileal pouch–anal anastomosis for UC. The aetiology of pouchitis is not well known, but bacteria are thought to play an important role, as confirmed by the great efficacy of antibiotic therapy.[30] Most patients have a relapsing disease, but in 15% this syndrome becomes a chronic disease that needs continued medical treatment with broad-spectrum antibiotics. In our study, 40 patients who were in clinical and endoscopic remission after 1 month of combined antibiotic treatment (rifaximin 2 g/day plus ciprofloxacin 1 g/day) were randomised to receive either VSL#3 6 g/day or an identical placebo for 9 months. Relapse was defined as an increase of at least two points in the clinical portion of PDAI (pouchitis disease activity index) and was confirmed by endoscopy and histology. Patients were assessed clinically every month, and endoscopically and histologically every 2 months or in case of relapse. Faecal samples, which were analysed for total aerobes and anaerobes, enterococci, bifidobacteria, lactobacilli, *Bacteroides, Clostridium* and coliforms, were collected at regular intervals. All 20 patients who received the placebo had a relapse. In contrast, 17 of 20 patients (85%) treated with VSL#3 were still in remission at the end of the study. Interestingly, all 17 patients relapsed within 4 months after stopping the active treatment. A significant increase in faecal concentrations of lactobacilli, bifidobacteria and *Streptococcus salivarius* subsp. *thermophilus* was found only in the VSL#3-treated group after 15 days of treatment, and was maintained throughout the study. This increase did not affect faecal concentrations of *Bacteroides,* coliforms, *Clostridium,* enterococci or total anaerobes and aerobes, strongly suggesting that the beneficial effect was not mediated by the suppression of endogenous flora.[31]

These positive effects of VSL#3 have been recently further confirmed in another double-blind, placebo-controlled study conducted to prevent pouchitis onset during the first year after pouch surgery. Forty patients, who underwent IPAA (ileal pouch-anal anastomosis) for UC were randomised to receive either VSL#3 3 g/day or an identical placebo for 12 months, within a week after ileostomy closure. Clinical, endoscopic and histological examinations were performed at 1, 3, 6, 9 and 12 months. Pouchitis was diagnosed according to the PDAI. Patients treated with VSL#3 had a significantly lower incidence of acute pouchitis (10%) than those treated with placebo (40%).[32]

Finally, we evaluated the efficacy and safety of a combined treatment consisting of a high dose of rifaximin (non-absorbable antibiotic) followed by VSL#3 versus mesalamine in the prevention of postoperative recurrence of Crohn's disease. Forty patients were randomised to receive, within a week after curative surgery, either rifaximin (1.8 g/day) for 3 months followed by VSL#3 (6 g/day) for 9 months, or mesalamine (4 g/day) for 12 months. Patients were assessed clinically and endoscopically at 3 and 12 months. At both 3 and 12 months patients treated with the combination of antibiotic and probiotic showed a significantly lower rate of severe endoscopic recurrence (10% and 20% vs. 40% and 40%; $P < 0.01$).[33]

With regard to the mechanism of action of VSL#3, we have demonstrated a significant increase in IL-10 tissue levels in patients with pouchitis during maintenance treatment.[34]

Conclusions

Many clinical and experimental observations suggest an involvement of the intestinal microflora in the pathogenesis of IBD. Highly concentrated probiotic preparations represent a valid approach for both the prevention of pouchitis onset and relapses. Whether the probiotic approach may also be effective for the treatment of CD and UC needs to be further assessed with large double-blind studies.

Future research should focus on obtaining more precise information on the composition of normal flora and on the mechanisms by which probiotic strains exert their beneficial effect to the host *in vivo*. This information will provide the scientific rationale for the choice of the best strains to conduct large controlled studies.

References

1. Bengmark S. Bacterial for optimal health. *Nutrition* 2000; 16:611–615.

2. Simon GL, Gorbach SL. Intestinal flora in health and disease. *Gastroenterology* 1984; 86:174–193.

3. Metchnikoff E. *The prolongation of life: optimistic studies.* In: Mitchell C, ed. *Prolongation of Life.* London: William Heinemann, 1907; 161–183.

4. Tissier H. Traitement des infections intestinales par la méthode de la flore bactérienne de l'intestin. *C Roy Soc Biol* 1906; 60:359–361.

5. Lilly DM, Stillwell RH. Probiotics: growth promoting factors produced by microorganisms. *Science* 1965; 47:747–748.

6. Fuller R. Probiotics in human medicine. *Gut* 1991; 32: 439–442.

7. Schaafsma G. State of the art concerning probiotic strains in milk products. *IDF Nutr Newslett* 1996; 5:23–24.

8. Lee YK, Salminen S. The coming age of probiotics. *Trends Food Sci Technol* 1995; 6: 241–245.

9. Wagner ED, Warner T, Roberts L, Farmer J, Balish E. Colonisation of congenitally immunodeficient mice with probiotic bacteria. *Infect Immunol* 1997; 65: 3345–3351.

10. Shanahan F. Therapeutic manipulation of gut flora. *Science* 2000; 289:1311–1312.

11. Sartor RB. Enteric microflora in IBD: pathogens or commensals? *Inflamm Bowel Dis* 1997; 3:230–235.

12. Duchmann R, Kaiser I, Hermann E, Mayet W, Ewe K, Meyer zum Buschenfelde K-H. Tolerance exists towards resident intestinal flora but is broken in active inflammatory bowel disease (IBD). *Clin Exp Immunol* 1995; 102:104–108.

13. MacPherson A, Khoo UY, Forgacs I, Philpott-Howard J, Bjarnason I. Mucosal antibodies in inflammatory bowel disease are directed against intestinal bacteria. *Gut* 1996; 38: 365–375.

14. Janpwitz HD, Croen EC, Sachar DB. The role of the faecal stream in Crohn's disease: an historical and analytic perspective. *Inflamm Bowel Dis* 1998; 4:29–39.

15. D'Haens GR, Geboes K, Peeters M, Penninckx F, Rutgeers SP. Early lesions of recurrent Crohn's disease caused by infusion of intestinal contents in excluded ileum. *Gastroenterology* 1998; 114:771–774.

16. Sartor RB. Insights into the pathogenesis of inflammatory bowel disease provided by new rodent models of spontaneous colitis. *Inflamm Bowel Dis* 1995; 1:64–75.

17. Campieri M, Gionchetti P. Probiotics in inflammatory bowel disease: new insight to pathogenesis or a possible therapeutic alternative? *Gastroenterology* 1999; 116: 1246–1249.

18. Fabia R, Ar'Rajab A, Johansson ML *et al.* Impairment of bacterial flora in human ulcerative colitis and experimental colitis in the rat. *Digestion* 1993; 54:248–255.

19. Favier C, Neut C, Mizon C, Cortot A, Colombel JF, Mizon J. Faecal ß-D-galactosidase production and bifidobacteria are decreased in Crohn's disease. *Dig Dis Sci* 1997; 42:817–822.

20. Ruseler-van-Embden JGH, Schouten WR, Van Lieshout LMC. Pouchitis: result of microbial imbalance? *Gut* 1994; 35:658–664.

21. Fabia R, Ar'rajab A, Johansson M-L, *et al.* The effect of exogenous administration of *Lactobacillus reuterii* R2LC and oat fibre on acetic acid-induced colitis in the rat. *Scand J Gastroenterol* 1993; 28:155–162.

22. Mao Y, Nobaek S, Kasravi B, *et al.* The effects of *Lactobacillus* strains and oat fibre on methotrexate-induced enterocolitis in rats. *Gastroenterology* 1996; 111:334–344.

23. Madsen KL, Tavernini MM, Doyle JSG, Fedorak RN. *Lactobacillus* sp prevents development of enterocolitis in interleukin-10 gene-deficient mice. *Gastroenterology* 1999; 116:1107–1114.

24. Schultz M, Veltkamp C, Dieleman LA, Wyrick PB, Tonkonogy SL, Sartor RB. Continuous feeding of *Lactobacillus plantarum* attenuates established colitis in interleukin-10 deficient mice. *Gastroenterology* 1998; 114: A1081.

25. Malchow HA. Crohn's disease and *Escherichia coli*. A new approach in therapy to maintain remission of colonic Crohn's disease? *J Clin Gastroenterol* 1997; 25: 653–658.

26. Kruis W, Schuts E, Fric P, Fixa B, Judmaier G, Stolte M. Double-blind comparison of an oral *Escherichia coli* preparation and mesalazine in maintaining remission of ulcerative colitis. *Aliment Pharmacol Ther* 1997; 11:853–858.

27. Rembacken BJ, Snelling AM, Hawkey P, Chalmers DM, Axon TR. Non pathogenic *Escherichia coli* vs mesalazine for the treatment of ulcerative colitis: a randomised trial. *Lancet* 1999; 354:635–639.

28. Guslandi M, Mezzi G, Sorghi M, *et al.* *Saccharomyces boulardii* in maintenance treatment of Crohn's disease. *Dig Dis Sci* 2000; 45:1462–1464.

29. Venturi A, Gionchetti P, Rizzello F, *et al.* Impact on the faecal flora composition of a new probiotic preparation. Preliminary data on maintenance treatment of patients with ulcerative colitis (UC) intolerant or allergic to 5-aminosalicylic acid (5 ASA). *Aliment Pharmacol Ther* 1999; 13:1103–1108.

30. Sartor RB. Probiotics in chronic pouchitis: restoring luminal microbial balance. *Gastroenterology* 2000; 119:584–585.

31. Gionchetti P, Rizzello F, Venturi A, *et al.* Oral bacteriotherapy as maintenance treatment in patients with chronic pouchitis: a double-blind, placebo-controlled trial. *Gastroenterology* 2000; 119:305–309.

32. Gionchetti P, Rizzello F, Venturi A, *et al.*. Profilaxis of pouchitis onset with probiotic therapy: a double blind, placebo-controlled trial. *Gastroenterology* 2000; 118:A190 [Abstract].

33. Campieri M, Rizzello F, Venturi A, *et al.* Combination of antibiotic and probiotic treatment is efficacious in prophylaxis of post-operative recurrence of Crohn's disease: a randomised controlled study vs. mesalazine. *Gastroenterology* 2000; 118:A781 [Abstract].

34. Gionchetti P, Rizzello F, Cifone G, *et al.* In vivo effect of a highly concentrated probiotic preparation on IL-10 pelvic ileal-pouch tissue levels. *Gastroenterology* 1999; 116:A723 [Abstract].

Summary and observations

Michael A Kamm

Substantial evidence has been cited throughout this book testifying to the fundamental role played by the gut flora in the development and maintenance of normal gut structure and function. Interactions between the host and microorganisms colonising the gut are prerequisites for normal gut motility, secretion, absorption, cell composition, mitotic activity, villous length and crypt depth. The normal flora also plays a key role in protecting against, or recovery from, enteric infections.

Despite this vast immunogenic reservoir, the maintenance of health and prevention of disease requires a finely tuned host immune system. Normal flora needs to be recognised and tolerated, and the presence of pathogens requires a sophisticated and aggressive, but limited, immune response.

Evidence has also been presented that the gut flora plays a central role in many gastrointestinal diseases. In addition to pathogenic enteric infections, the flora may play a role in conditions in which there is a loss of the normal tolerance to normal gut flora. Duchmann and co-workers have previously convincingly demonstrated that inflammatory bowel diseases are associated with loss of the normal tolerance to the normal indigenous gut flora.

The recent identification of variants of the *NOD2* gene as a predisposing factor for the development of Crohn's disease in about 20% of patients provides some basis for such a response. The protein encoded for by this gene is involved in bacterial detection and the subsequent inflammatory response. NOD2 seems to function as an intracellular receptor for lipopolysaccharide via a leucine-rich repeat domain (LRR), and is involved in the regulation of the NF-kB pathway, a key mediator of the genes involved in inflammation. This gene may confer susceptibility to Crohn's disease by altering the recognition of bacterial components, or by altering the activation of NF-kB in immune cells.

An abnormal response to normal, or abnormal, gut flora is also a prime suspect in a number of extraintestinal disorders, such as atopy, the spectrum of autoimmune disorders, and arthritis.

Given the weight of evidence supporting a central role for the gut flora in maintaining health, and in promoting a number of diseases, the possibility of modifying this internal environment to prevent disease or restore health is tantalising. Sound clinical controlled evidence is now emerging to support such an approach.

The greatest body of evidence for modifying the gut flora currently relates to the ingestion of probiotic bacteria, that is, bacteria which confer health benefits or disease-modifying characteristics in excess of their nutritional value. Classically, various types of lactobacilli and bifidobacteria have been considered to have such properties, although even within these species the evidence for therapeutic benefit varies between strains. Other bacteria, such as certain strains of *Escherichia coli* have also been shown to have therapeutic value.

Erika Isolauri summarises some of the evidence for benefit of probiotic ingestion in conditions of gastrointestinal infection, and in some extraintestinal childhood conditions. Probiotic bacteria may have a role in preventing and attenuating rotavirus infection. Other evidence attests to the value of probiotic bacteria in preventing antibiotic-associated diarrhoea and in the treatment of recurrent *Clostridium difficile* infection.

The ability of probiotic bacteria to improve the course of atopic eczema in infants raises many questions about the possible mode of action of such a therapy:

· Do these organisms contribute to the repair of a defective epithelial barrier, thereby decreasing systemic exposure to enteral antigens?
· Do they activate epithelial cells or epithelial immune cells in a way which diminishes an abnormal response to enteral commensals?
· Do they diminish the presence of specific strains of bacteria that drive this inflammatory disorder?

These are just some of the possible mechanisms that require investigation.

Recent studies from Isolauri and colleagues have shown that infants who go on to develop an atopic diathesis have a different luminal chemical milieu, with associated differences from normal in the proportion of various identifiable gut bacteria. Furthermore, the administration of probiotic bacteria appears to reduce the development of an atopic condition. These fascinating studies should encourage us to explore this therapeutic approach in the vast range of non-gastrointestinal disorders which may have an underlying antigenic drive as their pathogenic basis, such as the autoimmune and arthritic diseases.

Returning to disorders of the gut, it is perhaps easiest in this setting to appreciate the potential benefit for modification of the bacterial environment. In the inflammatory bowel diseases the administration of probiotic bacteria have started to have a real therapeutic impact. Campieri, Gionchetti and colleagues have shown in controlled trials that the administration of a concentrated mixture of multiple strains of probiotic bacteria will maintain remission in patients with an ileoanal reservoir in whom antibiotics have healed an acute episode of inflammation (pouchitis), and prevent pouchitis when administered prophylactically. Both the antibiotic healing of the acute inflammation and the maintenance of a healthy mucosa by altering the luminal milieu, form convincing evidence for the primary role of bacteria in driving the inflammatory process in this condition. This group has also shown a decreased endoscopic recurrence in postoperative patients with Crohn's disease given antibiotics and probiotics after curative resection.

A number of groups have shown that various *Escherichia coli* strains are equally effective as mesalazine in preventing relapse in patients with ulcerative colitis. These studies have employed low doses of mesalazine or have had unexpectedly high relapse rates in both treatment groups, making the interpretation of these studies uncertain. This is well described in the chapter by Gionchetti and colleagues.

Evidence is beginning to emerge which defines the mechanisms underlying these clinical findings. Probiotic bacteria have been shown to colonise the gut during therapy and to induce specific pH and other chemical changes in the lumen. The immune changes induced by these bacteria are also coming under scrutiny. Animal studies have highlighted some of the modifying properties of these bacteria. Our own group has shown differences in the cytokine response of human dendritic cells – the earliest cells involved in bacterial antigen recognition – to different probiotic bacteria.

These are early days. The therapeutic road of manipulating the gut bacterial environment is one of enormous potential, made even more attractive by the aesthetic appeal of such a natural, and apparently safe, approach. In his concluding remarks, Fergus Shanahan has highlighted some of the many questions that need to be addressed in these therapies. These range from the need for controlled trials with different organisms, doses and combinations of organisms, to studying their mode of action. The number of conditions in which they may find a role is great. Once their mechanism has been defined, more intriguing questions will emerge about the biochemical nature of the bacterial–epithelial, bacterial–immune, and bacterial–bacterial interactions. These questions hold the key to identifying new classes of substances that mediate these effects. Molecular tools will be of central importance in opening up this treasure chest.

Index